Elizabeth Bryan and
Ronald Higgins

Infertility

NEW CHOICES, NEW DILEMMAS

PENGUIN BOOKS

PENGUIN BOOKS

Published by the Penguin Group
Penguin Books Ltd, 27 Wrights Lane, London w8 5tz, England
Penguin Books USA Inc., 375 Hudson Street, New York, New York 10014, USA
Penguin Books Australia Ltd, Ringwood, Victoria, Australia
Penguin Books Canada Ltd, 10 Alcorn Avenue, Toronto, Ontario, Canada m4v 3b2
Penguin Books (NZ) Ltd, 182–190 Wairau Road, Auckland 10, New Zealand

Penguin Books Ltd, Registered Offices: Harmondsworth, Middlesex, England

First published 1995
1 3 5 7 9 10 8 6 4 2

Set in 10.5/13pt Monotype Sabon
Typeset by Datix International Limited, Bungay, Suffolk
Printed in England by Clays Ltd, St Ives plc

Contents

Introduction

This book arose from the pain of our own infertility, our dogged hopes of finding a remedy and our experience of both frustration and partial compensation for our childlessness. In it we describe the historical background to infertility as well as its physiology, but our emphasis is on the many wider, controversial issues stemming from the profound revolution in reproductive technologies that are still developing at a rapid rate. After explaining many new reproductive technologies and their sometimes bewildering implications, we look especially at the new choices and dilemmas they are throwing up, not only for would-be parents and the medical professionals who care for them but for society at large.

The book therefore attempts to deal with these issues as the necessary concern of everyone – not least as citizens, voters and taxpayers – as well as providing a general guide to subfertile couples, who may be grappling with the new possibilities and procedures for the first time, and offering a useful overview for medical professionals. These are not conflicting aims. The general reader needs to appreciate the special pains of involuntary childlessness but, equally, the couple seeking treatment may find it helpful to explore the many wider significances of what they are undertaking.

Since we are addressing several different audiences at once, we must therefore expect certain readers to skip, say, some of the physiological description while others skim over the discussion of the latest legal changes. But, this said, we have been intrigued to find how many subjects must come into any overall view of infertility and its remedies. Questions of physiology, endocrinology, medical practice, history, myth, philosophy, psychology, ethics, law, demography and, not least, health policy, economics and politics – even world politics – are encompassed. For the non-medical reader the Glossary at the end of the book will provide help with some of the technical terms associated with infertility and its treatment.

Neither of the authors is involved with the provision of infertility diagnosis or treatment. Elizabeth Bryan is a consultant paediatrician, founder and medical director of the Multiple Births Foundation (MBF) and author of several books on the nature and nurture of twins, triplets and higher multiple births – the number of which is rising at a worrying rate as a result of some infertility treatments being employed injudiciously. She has organized many study days concerning infertility treatment and has lectured widely on its possible repercussions. Since 1991 she has also acted as one of the official inspectors of British infertility clinics, appointed by the Human Fertilisation and Embryology Authority (HFEA).

Ronald Higgins is a former diplomat and journalist with interests in global environmental issues, not least those of population, but increasingly in the psychological, social and ethical aspects of public health. He once directed the Richmond Fellowship's national network of therapeutic communities for the mentally ill and has contributed to various medical publications. He is chairman of the Champernowne Trust for Psychotherapy and, since 1991, a non-executive director and vice-chairman of the Herefordshire Community Health NHS Trust.

Both of us write here in a personal capacity; our views are not necessarily shared by the institutions which we serve. We are both committed to the fullest public discussion of all the delicate and often controversial aspects of this fascinating subject. Throughout a necessarily wide-ranging debate of the social implications we hope sight will never be lost of the sometimes desperate needs of the infertile, whether in success or failure.

While neither of us has experience of giving, rather than receiving, infertility treatment, we take comfort in the thought that no one can be an expert in all the aspects we have covered here. What we have attempted to convey is a comprehensive overview, the details of which have been checked by several specialists in the areas least familiar to us. Nevertheless we take full responsibility for any errors or omissions that may remain.

The book would not have been written without the help of many other minds and hands. We cannot thank everyone but must mention the particular gratitude we owe to Jane Denton, Alison Elliman, Peter Foot, Flora Goldhill, Faith Hallett, Mary Lister, Bridget Mason and Lalage Neal. In addition we especially thank Jane Gardiner for her consistently cheerful help with the manuscripts and Ivor Badham for carrying them across our valley to and from Jane, in fine weather and in foul. Many thanks are also due to the medical professionals of all kinds whom we have met privately or at professional conferences, at home and abroad. Carol Heaton, friend as well as literary agent, had the idea for this book and has been marvellously encouraging throughout. Finally we are grateful to its editor and contributors for permission to quote from the, often anonymous, articles in *Prospect Newsletter*, published by Prospect, the IVF Unit, Hammersmith Hospital, London.

This book is dedicated to Margaret Beall, Elizabeth's godmother. Although without children herself, her warmth, enthusiasm and generosity have enriched the lives of countless children.

1. The Reproductive Revolution . . . and One Couple's Story

In our world of rapid change there have been many revolutions but few so profound as that which has taken place in the field of human reproduction.

The Cold War has ended and the revival of ancient conflicts has caused the world's maps to be redrawn. The widening gulf between the rich and poor is creating new problems. Most homes in the well-off industrialized countries now have not only a car and all sorts of household machinery but a robot-made television set bringing instantaneous news from across a globe that, within living memory, used to take many months to circumnavigate. In industry, the production of armaments, modes of communication and entertainment there has probably been more change in the past hundred years than in the previous two thousand. Nevertheless the medical capacities developed in only the last two decades have brought about a yet more profound transformation – one concerning the ways our children may now be conceived, gestated and brought to birth.

The new methodologies are capable not only of overcoming or circumventing many of the most serious problems of the infertile but of providing unprecedented possibilities for the pre-selection of sperm and eggs, and indeed for their manipulation. Some people are presenting the revolution in a highly dramatic form. They say we started by separating sex from reproduction by using birth control. Now we are separating procreation from sex by using laboratory dishes, and parenting from genetics by using donated sperm or eggs. We can even separate parenting from pregnancy by employing surrogate mothers.

A woman can now have a child by someone she has never met. Women who are well past menopause, sixty years old or more, have already produced 'test-tube' babies. It may even become technically possible for men to sustain a pregnancy (and deliver by a Caesarean section). There is now no extrinsic technical difficulty about producing babies from sperm, eggs or both from donors who are dead – so-called posthumous procreation. Controversies have also been burning fiercely about the morality of making up the shortage of donated eggs by taking them from the bodies of dead women or even, in the future, aborted fetuses.

The new techniques have already enabled embryos to be frozen and brought to birth several years later and at different times, so that one twin can be gestated and born years after the other one. In theory the new techniques also allow a couple to choose both eggs and sperm from a preferred donor and have the resulting embryo brought to birth by a surrogate mother so that their own busy lives can proceed uninterrupted.

The new methods of assisted conception open up other dramatic scenarios. Embryologists can already detect, avoid using or remove some of the egg's genes that carry menacing diseases, and may be able to achieve much more as they progressively unravel the genetic strands of life. They may become technically – if also very controversially – able to satisfy some would-be parents' demands concerning their children's gender, race and likely appearance and, in due course, even their talents and temperament.

While some of these medical dreams seem more like nightmares, many may prove impracticable as well as unethical. Some of the new techniques may disgust us but gradually become acceptable when the benefits to the infertile are more widely appreciated. After all, organ transplants, even blood transfusions, were once thought an intolerable interference in the natural order of things.

As always in the human story, new technological capabilities produce new choices and dilemmas. Many of the current infertility treatments have been gratefully welcomed by would-be parents, but where should the limits lie? Can we fulfil the longings of the childless without slithering down the perilous slopes that so many media articles are warning us about?

Infertility and subfertility are subjects of such sensitivity, moral complexity and practical significance that the reader deserves to know something of the background of both authors: our relevant experiences and any limitations. First, then, we must describe the discovery of our own infertility and what happened as each of us saw it.

Elizabeth's Story

I am told that I was six when I first announced that I would be a children's doctor, not because I particularly yearned to be a doctor but because I wanted to work with children. I always loved young children. As a teenager I spent many happy days organizing children's parties and even the pony club's under-fives, in whom no serious horse rider was ever interested. Later I took infinite pleasure in my many godchildren. They would come for an annual week-long camp in the orchard of my cottage high on the North York moors. Children have always been at the centre of my life and it never occurred to me that I should not have as many as I wanted when I wanted them.

When I met and married Ronald in 1978, we assumed that children would naturally follow and become part of our life together. I was thirty-six and Ronald forty-nine. In view of our ages we decided it would be better not to delay. Assuming we would conceive as soon as we tried, we took precautions for the first three months while we settled into our new home. This now seems ironic and I still deeply regret missing those first opportunities.

For the next three months the arrival of my monthly period brought disappointment but not distress. After six months I became increasingly worried. My family doctor was reassuring and helpful. Realizing that time was not on our side, he examined me and arranged a sperm count for Ronald. We were both intensely relieved when this was found to be normal. Yet my own situation was still in question, or there could be some sort of incompatibility even if we were both fertile.

Just after our first wedding anniversary my usually mechanically regular period was late and I felt sick, although this may have been from a sense of anticipation. Two weeks later my home-kit pregnancy test showed the vital positive blue ring. We were overjoyed. We had never concealed the fact that we were trying hard for a baby, and soon our families and friends were sharing our happiness. Because we were such late starters, most of our friends had older children and they too were excited for us. We were very touched by the general delight.

Even before our pregnancy we had clear ideas about how children were to fit into our lives and ours into theirs. Ronald and I would each work part-time and share the care. We both therefore entered the pregnancy with deep interest and excitement. I felt well but just nauseated enough to reassure me that I was pregnant. Our local hospital was a large teaching hospital and I registered there after eight weeks and was disappointed that I had to wait another month before having an ultrasound scan. I was longing to see my baby.

The next two weeks went by happily but I had an almost unacknowledged worry that I was not 'feeling' more pregnant. I no longer felt sick in the morning and the tension in my breasts had decreased. Then, one evening, after returning from the theatre, I discovered some faint brown staining. I knew this was blood. My heart sank and I went to bed. The next morning I saw the doctor and was told to stay in bed. The following day I began to get cramps in my stomach, and when the doctor gave me an internal examination, he found that the pregnancy was over. My baby had never started to develop: I had a 'blighted ovum'. For the next twenty-four hours I lay in bed with increasingly severe stomach cramps and intermittently wept, as did Ronald, for the loss of our precious baby. I did not grieve the loss of motherhood. It did not occur to me that I would have any difficulty getting pregnant again. We had managed once; we would manage again.

Our friends and family shared our sadness and were tremendously supportive. I was glad we had been so open about our pregnancy. Their sympathy was wonderful and most of them continued to help us throughout our long saga of infertility.

I impatiently waited for the statutory three months advised by the doctor to pass, and then we tried again. Over the next six months there were several times when I felt pregnant but each came to nothing. My obstetrician examined me carefully and found nothing wrong. With our encouragement, however, he agreed to start tests straight away. So began the round of X-rays, ultrasound scans, salpingogram, tubal insufflation, post-coital tests. Much of our life was now dominated by my temperature chart. Not only did it dictate our pattern of love-making but that of our working life too. I worked mostly in London, Ronald in Herefordshire, so we would normally have been apart for several nights each week. Even the most important engagements now had to be changed, or even missed, if they meant our being in different beds during the crucial time.

Each test brought with it the reassuring news that we were 'normal' but also the disappointment that there was nothing therefore to treat.

Meanwhile my younger sister, Felicity, also in her later thirties, had a daughter and a son in quick succession, followed by another son. Bernadette, six years younger, had two daughters in 1985 and 1988. Felicity's first child was conceived in 1981 at the first attempt. Until then I had been lucky in not suffering much jealousy at the good fortune of my friends, partly perhaps because most of them had completed their families some years before. The main problem I had to cope with was their embarrassment as they tried to hide from me their excitement about a forthcoming grandchild or the news of a termination for an unplanned 'afterthought'.

However, the arrival of babies in my own family proved harder to take than I had expected. My sisters were enormously sensitive to my feelings but there was nothing they could do to reduce my envy or ease my longing as I watched the infinite pleasure the children gave to their parents and grandparents.

My fortieth birthday was now rapidly approaching. Our anxiety increased as we realized that time was running out. Friends, including many medical ones, bombarded us with suggestions for increasing our fertility. We considered each idea seriously. It was said I was 'working too hard', so I went to bed for a week each month. After three months I abandoned this very inconvenient practice. We were now apparently 'trying too hard'. The temperature charts were thrown away and I tried not to count the days. It was impossible. One friend, with some embarrassment, suggested my thyroid gland could be the problem. More tests were conducted, which again proved negative.

For six months I tried a weekly one-hour session of acupuncture in north London. This sometimes involved a special journey from our home in Herefordshire, 150 miles away. It was even a good hour's journey from my London office. Whether or not the acupuncture would result in our having a baby, I felt it was well worthwhile. Amid all the tests and treatments this was the first time I had felt cared for as a person. No longer was it just the functioning of my various gynaecological and endocrinological parts that were of interest but my whole being, physical and emotional. I looked forward to my acupuncture sessions. Sometimes I felt strange immediately afterwards, but usually I felt more relaxed and stronger. Yet there was still no sign of a pregnancy.

I have believed in the power of faith healing since I was a

child. My grandmother used to visit a faith healer and I saw how she received remarkable relief from her long-standing arthritis. So when a friend I greatly respect suggested a trip to a faith healer in Dundee, Ronald and I set off in an optimistic frame of mind for a weekend in Scotland.

The healer had an unusual background. Formerly an army officer's wife and ardent follower of foxhounds, she suddenly discovered her powers of healing in late middle age and at once put these to generous and beneficial use. Hers was a Christian form of faith healing but she also incorporated other techniques, including pendulum swinging and Bach flower remedies.

I came away feeling uplifted and more at peace but having been recommended to follow a most tiresome diet: the pendulum swinging over my body had indicated an allergy to aluminium. All cooking utensils containing aluminium were sent off to the next jumble sale. Friends were asked not to cook in such pans or use foil. It was surprising we received any invitations to eat out at all.

As the months passed and the frustrations mounted, my religious faith wavered. At times I became very angry. I felt God had misled me. Why should I have been given such an instinctive love for children and apparent gifts for relating to them if I was not to be allowed any of my own? In addition I found the uncertainty almost the hardest part to bear. For a person who was a great planner (to a fault, some would say) and who assumed her plans would work out, I found the uncertainty of not knowing what would be happening to us next month, let alone next year, very difficult to cope with.

Meanwhile, on the orthodox medical front, the full battery of relevant tests were completed and had still revealed nothing abnormal. We were classified as a case of 'unexplained infertility' and, because I was now forty, we were told nothing more could be done.

It was only four years since Louise Brown, the first 'test-tube' baby, had been born. In vitro fertilization (IVF) and the other new reproductive technologies were in their infancy and the success rates were still low. For those over forty they were very low indeed. I already knew that my specialist would not consider entering me into such a programme. The waiting list was several years long, in any case.

I therefore approached the department at the hospital where I work myself and, as it happened, the only one at the time that had a National Health Service programme for IVF. After yet another series of tests, all of which proved normal, it was agreed that we should be allowed one attempt at IVF. We knew that our chances of success were small, but if they had been only one in a hundred – perhaps even one in a thousand – I think I would still have wanted to have a go, not least to convince ourselves that we had tried everything. I did not want to be haunted ever afterwards by the thought 'if only'. If we attempted IVF and failed, we should at least know there was no realistic hope of ever having our own child, and the uncertainty would be over.

We entered the programme immediately and within about two months were offered our first and only attempt. In those days there was no routine counselling, but an enthusiastic registrar encouraged us as best he could as he hurried along the row of candidates anxiously awaiting their blood tests and ultrasound scans. The order and timing of events that month are now a blur but some of the experiences remain vivid in my mind.

One of my few good memories was the amazing camaraderie of the ten women who were facing the 'challenge' of IVF treatment that month. We had come from all over the world. A few, like me, were on their first attempt and were hugely grateful for the guidance of the more experienced.

It was like an endurance test with predictable times of crisis. Some of us would drop out because our ovaries failed to respond to the stimulation of the hormone injections; others when eggs were not retrieved; more if the eggs failed to fertilize; a last group if none of their embryos became implanted in the womb. We all understood it was unlikely that more than one, or possibly two, of us would end up with a baby, and no one could know who that would be.

The suspense was intense as we sat with our bladders full to bursting waiting for our ultrasound scans. The verdict would decide whether we could go forward to the next stage, the retrieval of the eggs. Failure at any stage brought despair and often anger for the candidate concerned, but enormous sympathy from the rest of us.

Egg retrieval in those days was conducted under general anaesthetic, for me an ordeal as I am always horribly sick afterwards. But we were lucky: four eggs were retrieved and Ronald and I were overjoyed. (Only one of our group fell at this hurdle.) Then Ronald had to drive up quickly from Herefordshire during the night to produce the fresh semen needed for the attempted IVF.

By now only three of us were in synchrony: others were a day or two ahead or behind. We three then supported each other over the telephone as we anxiously waited for the requisite forty-eight hours to pass to hear whether any of our eggs had been fertilized.

If all four of our eggs were fertilized, Ronald and I would have to decide how many of them should be implanted. We were told there would be a slightly greater chance of having one baby if all four embryos were used. But that would necessarily mean some chance of having more than one baby. We discussed at length whether it would be right to risk giving birth to quadruplets. (In those days there were no restrictions on how many embryos could be transferred.) Ronald said he was happy to leave the decision to me. I had few doubts that quads would be better than no child at all. If all the eggs were fertilized, we would therefore ask to have all four transferred.

I am grateful that I had the opportunity to face this dilemma myself, however briefly, because it has helped to convince me that few couples undergoing the emotional strain of infertility treatment would be able to make an objective decision. I now realize that, for us, quads would not have been a happy outcome, and not for the children either.

The forty-eight hours crept past, and after a night of sleepless suspense, I rang in at the allotted hour and was disappointed to hear that only one of our eggs had been fertilized. At least we had one fertilized egg, though, with no risk of producing quads. But the chance of a pregnancy was now very low indeed.

Together with the other members of our trio, I was readmitted to hospital for the embryo transfer. Once in the operating theatre, I was allowed to look at my embryo – a few transparent, but live, cells under the microscope. It was the most exciting moment of all. Never have I had a more precious sight and one in which such hope had been invested. I shall never forget it.

After a night in hospital, I returned home to Herefordshire having been assured that if my embryo was strong enough to become implanted, it would do so on its own and there was no way I could help it by, for instance, lying head downwards or even staying in bed for several days. I tried to get on with ordinary life, but it was impossible. I could think of nothing except whether my period would or would not appear in a few days' time. The first possible day came and went, and the second and the third. But by the fourth there were unmistakeable feelings of premenstrual tension, and sure enough the first spotting appeared that day. That was the end of my quest for a baby.

I do not know what happened to my two friends. Despite our good intentions, we did not get in touch again. Perhaps none of us could bear to face the success of the others. Perhaps we were too preoccupied with our own grief, and then it seemed too late to regain contact.

In the following days Ronald and I talked about adoption but, perhaps surprisingly, both of us agreed quite quickly not even to explore that route. We knew that we would both be considered too old to adopt a healthy baby through any official agencies. (I was actually the medical adviser to an adoption agency at the time and knew the rules only too well.)

Even if a healthy baby could have been made available to us, I rather doubt that either of us would have wanted to proceed. Despite my longing for a child, I felt that if we were not able to have one ourselves, particularly when there was no obvious medical impediment, then our childlessness was somehow meant to be. Perhaps our lives were destined to go in a different direction – although I did not find this easy to accept at the time.

Nevertheless the destruction of our long-standing hopes felt like a terrible bereavement, which proved to be long and painful. Several years on, we still feel a sense of loss and sometimes a new setback arises. For instance, the birth of a close friend's first grandchild finally brought home to us the fact that we would never experience that special joy ourselves. We were similarly affected by the arrival of the first baby born to one of my godchildren. I still think about my own child, the one who miscarried at ten weeks, and what she (somehow I know she was a girl) would – should – have been doing now, thirteen years later. I do sometimes resent the fact that, in the long subsequent story of our infertility, people have forgotten, however understandably, our own short-lived pregnancy and the child it represented.

I have learned how to cope with the feeling of loss most of the time. Moments of overwhelming sadness are rare although some events, such as christenings, are always an ordeal for us. Yet, looking back and imagining if we had had a child or children, I doubt that I would have had the time and energy to create the Multiple Births Foundation. We certainly would not have gained the necessary experience from which to write this book. Undoubtedly there have been compensations. I accept that my life may be as rich without our own children. I would still never have chosen that it should be that way.

Ronald's Story

Perhaps like most men, I always assumed I should eventually have children. It would be a natural part of marriage, a natural part of life, a natural continuation of the family relationships I had enjoyed in my youth. My mother had been one of four, with five half-brothers and sisters. My father had been one of thirteen.

Whether I 'wanted' children, as opposed to expected them, is a more complex question. I would probably not have volunteered for fatherhood. Neither in my youth nor my early adulthood did I find babies interesting or attractive. Nor did my pulse beat any faster at the sight of a baby. If it was crying, I retreated as quickly as any of my sex. Babies were apparently a necessary stage in the production of children, and the sooner the baby grew into a child, the better.

Not that I was positively keen on children, either. Taken singly, they could be demanding; taken in groups, they could be deafening. For anyone preoccupied by his work or hobbies, especially reading or music, any child was a distraction at best, a destroyer at worst.

Children also needed washing, clothing, feeding, housing and even care and attention. I had no objection to any creatures, including sheep, poultry and cattle, receiving their own due nurturing. It was just that I felt no especial desire to farm the stock in question, let alone sire it. Having children plainly meant paying an immense price in time, ease of life and money: I detected no great urge in myself deliberately to incur such obligations. I generously acknowledged that the human race had to be perpetuated but did not think my own genes were likely to make any especially necessary contribution.

By my late twenties I began to see children as potentially attractive. Not my own: I was yet to acquire a permanent partner, let alone start a family. But when friends showed clear delight in their recognizably individual progeny, I was bound to take some interest. Suspicion had already been replaced by neutrality; now emerged a cautious regard. It might, after all, be nice to have children, and not just accept Nature and Inevitability!

I was married for the first time at thirty-six but was promptly whisked off by the Diplomatic Service to an Indonesia with which Britain was effectively at war and where the Embassy had recently been burned to the ground. Survival seemed a wiser immediate aim than procreation. Nor did my then wife, a dedicated and ambitious journalist, feel any urgent desire to start a family. Until we parted five years later, we concentrated on our professional lives.

Only when I married Elizabeth (Libby) many years later did the wish for children become real. The unqualified strength of her own desire for children was hugely impressive, and I found myself quite simply wanting it to be fulfilled. Approaching fifty, I had also by then become acquainted with one or two children myself.

That may sound extraordinary but perhaps many adults, especially men, may never get to know a child, let alone watch him or her develop. There may be no candidates in their family or other close circle. I had, however, recently been lucky. After my divorce I had bought a weekend cottage on the Welsh border, and a small bright girl called Vicky, who lived nearby with her grandparents, often came to chat and even help with the weeding. She was a dear child and a passionate learner. Despite being a somewhat gruff and morose recluse at that time, I found her enthusiasm, intelligence and sense of humour heart-warming. Over the many years she lived nearby, Vicky taught me more than I taught her and now, nearly twenty years later, flourishes in her profession.

When, therefore, I married for the second time, the idea of having children was no longer abstract or routine. There was a desire for my own version of my first child-friend and, above all, for an already deeply happy marriage to Libby to be completed. The idea of children bearing resemblance to both of us was at once moving, mysterious and comical. I laughed, and later cried, at the thought.

The arrival of children would plainly greatly complicate our busy working and social lives. For both of us they would represent a radical departure from what we were used to. As my work was more static and less hectically demanding than a consultant paediatrician's, much of the parenting would fall to me. The arrival of a child would therefore present an ominous challenge not only to my treasured solitude but to my wholly untried capacities for nurturing. Libby said I should play at least an equal part. I could see the fairness in this, even if the thought made me tremble.

As she has said, we delayed our first attempts to conceive a child. I was not myself sorry. The idea of children is one thing; their imminent arrival quite another. But in our case that prospect gradually receded.

I was relieved, perhaps disproportionately, that my sperm count proved to be within the normal range and that nothing wrong was found in Libby. The months passed and then, just a year from our wedding, we had managed it. Libby was pregnant. And a few weeks later, suddenly, she was not.

My most vivid memory of that time in our life was Libby's expression when she realized she had lost the baby. I had turned instinctively towards her and saw at once that her face had drained. It had the look of death on it: she seemed to be gazing into some awful black chasm. I gasped at the pain and we fell together, without words, in tears.

Whether I have ever fully digested the horror of that night

or wholly faced our childlessness, I cannot be sure. I believe I largely have, but the process may have been slower and less conscious in me than in Libby. I still cry readily at the grief of others.

Following this failure, the next stages of the medical investigation mostly involved Libby alone. Some of the less orthodox practitioners were, however, interested in the quality of our relationship and therefore wanted to see both of us. I felt no problem with this, but rather welcomed it. Fertility and infertility had not only a clinical, physiological side but surely also psychological and spiritual aspects in which we are all novices. But even had I been utterly sceptical about these matters, I know that for Libby's sake I would have suspended disbelief and tried virtually anything.

Sometimes both of us were tense with apprehension. New hopes were soon succeeded by new disappointments; bright new avenues led into new frustrations. We were lucky to be able to express our see-sawing emotions to each other, however discreditable or ungrateful these night-time feelings sometimes looked in the cold dawn, or the warm sunshine.

We needed to be very patient with each other: the strains often told on us. Some of the medical practitioners were maddeningly cool and mechanical. Some of the less orthodox ones we visited were vague and pretentious, their arcane methods seeming at times to border on the superstitious. I was often affronted by their woolly language, dubious assumptions and probably untestable claims. But infertility seemed a mysterious business: we still had no diagnosis and no dependable hope. Some things in medicine work even where there is no clear theory to go with them.

Nor was it easy for me, any more than for Libby, to make love on the dictates of a thermometer. It did not prove physically difficult but it was upsetting to do on instruction what we had previously done only through desire or impulse. It was sometimes hard to sustain our confidence in the thought that all the rearrangements, disturbances and sudden journeys would prove worthwhile. But somehow, when our hopes fluctuated, we had to boost each other's morale and hence determination to see the matter through. About Libby's resolution I had no doubt: it seemed unshakeable. All I needed to do was to fit in with whatever each new stage demanded.

This sometimes brought with it high costs, literal and metaphorical. We could not organize either work or play with anything like our normal flexibility. At times it felt as if our sole conversational subject was how to achieve our only serious objective: our child. We earned less, produced less and often disappointed our families and friends with seemingly erratic changes of plan. They were mostly very patient and considerate with us: fortunately we felt able to explain to nearly all of them just why it was sometimes so difficult to get hold of us or to pin down a particular date for meeting up.

There was still, I must confess, an element of ambivalence in me about having children: success meant at once what I wanted and what in part I still feared. I did not believe I should regret parenthood once achieved, but many unknowns remained. This is not the best mental condition to be in when one's partner is experiencing either dreadful fears or intoxicating hopes. Nevertheless I found Libby's single-minded longing for a child, our child, inexpressibly moving: my shaky confidence was often restored by hers.

The many doctors and nurses we met were primarily concerned with the mystery of our difficulties in conceiving, but most of them proved to be carefully considerate throughout the many explanations and procedures, not least in treating us as a couple.

At our infertility clinic I saw less of the men than Libby saw of the women. Yet I still vividly and affectionately recall the gentle giant from Nigeria and the lively lawyer from the Gulf States. When the nurse seemed vague about exactly where I should leave my (numbered but not named) phial of semen, I found myself wondering which of us would end up siring whose child.

The events of that time are now a blur of waiting rooms and midnight cross-country drives to the clinic, where I would find Libby looking pale and tired but brave as she faced the next test, procedure or disappointment. To me little but her health and morale and, only then, a successful result seemed to matter.

Libby has told what happened with our one permitted attempt at IVF. That period was sometimes hectic, sometimes exciting, sometimes tedious, and often miserable. When finally we had failed, I felt relief that the switchback emotions of hope, despair and suspense were over. But I had to go at Libby's own emotional pace. I waited quietly for her to work through her own feelings although I felt immense gratitude when she bravely decided that a baby was not to be and that she would therefore herself call a halt to the otherwise endless oscillation of hope and frustration. She just cut her losses. Her decisiveness frankly shocked me. But life became easier for us both. I am still puzzled that she could so decide to change course. And I am still profoundly grateful for the courage she showed.

As the years have passed, we have often talked about the family we never had, but about the benefits as well as the sadnesses of childlessness. When on the spur of the moment we decide to spend an evening at the theatre or a weekend in the Welsh mountains, we can mostly do just that. Indeed we have been on long lecture tours in Japan and Australia without having to worry about anything more than our pockets and our respective performances. This is not the alleged selfishness of the childless: we could hardly have done more to generate the pitter-patter of tiny feet. Our task has changed: it has become one of making something good, both at work and play, out of the eventual failure of what had been our paramount hope.

Our ultimate disappointment was intense. The whole saga

had been an ordeal for us both; we were emotionally exhausted. But our pain was nothing compared with that of many. We were relatively old when we married, so we had already had to consider the possibility of not having children. We were always able to talk freely to each other, and to other people. We had family, friends and colleagues who were endlessly generous in their support. We suffered little frustration from unsympathetic or uncomprehending medical professionals, or from long waiting lists. We understood the biology. We had no great moral doubts. We did not undergo the financial strains of repeated expensive treatments.

We are glad that we tried hard, and remain profoundly grateful to those who helped us, not least other patients, some of whom went through much crueller times. Gradually over the years we have tried to find ways to use our experience positively. Perhaps this book may prove to be one of these.

2. Myths, Motives and the New Opportunities

Until the last century most talk about the begetting of children would have been laced with superstition, old wives' tales, magic potions, curses and the interpretation of dreams. Now it is increasingly concerned with subtleties in medical diagnosis and new tricks performed in the laboratory and clinic. But the old ideas retain some power, at least over our emotions, so our thinking about infertility needs to bridge both worlds: that of age-old images and feelings, and that of contemporary medicine.

Psychologists describe the first as a realm of profound instincts, unconscious impulses and, for some, of subterranean longings, dark fears and burning hopes. The second is governed by scientific objectivity, technical ingenuity, disciplined routines and the 'can-do' optimism of modern culture. Both these perspectives deserve respect. One of them may well determine our deepest personal feelings and responses, and the other the practical outcome of long and perhaps stressful processes.

There are few areas of medicine where understanding the particular patient, and her or his partner, is more vital. Sometimes the obstacle to a successful pregnancy is obvious. But even where the diagnosis is straightforward, there may be a hidden load of fear and anxiety in one or both partners. No infertility treatment, however simple, is just a matter of 'getting mended'.

Our hunger for children and urge to nurture them are evidenced every day through tales of baby-snatching, baby-smuggling and phantom pregnancies. The longing for them is deeply rooted in our biological nature but also our cultural history. The symbolic force of ideas about fertility in particular is apparent in our ancient myths. Possibly the most popular of all Greek goddesses was Artemis who, like her Roman counterpart, Diana, was at once a goddess of wild creatures and the chase, and a fertility deity who aided both conception and childbirth.

Some dismiss these myths as mildly amusing vestiges of a primitive past with no bearing on the problems of today's patients. But such associations of maternity with Mother Earth and of fertility with creativity may well affect, and perhaps help, an infertile couple in their attitudes, choices and even their response to treatment. All sorts of longings, fears, cultural traditions and personal experiences accompany the apprehensive couple as they come through the clinic door. Each of them has their own story to tell. Medicine has to respond to the whole person and therefore all the powerful feelings and ideas, rational or not, with which the patient arrives.

In the briskly wide-awake, secular world of the modern metropolis we can be tempted to dismiss any suggestions of connections between our own fertility and that of the earth around us. Women, and men too, can be taken aback by powerful feelings, awesome dreams or seemingly irrational impulses. Some ancient ideas or symbols can have a modern relevance, if only in making some sense of unexpected experiences.

The Tree of Life

Many societies have always perceived a 'magic' two-way relationship between fertility in woman and fertility in crops. Bavarian and Austrian peasants, for instance, will give the first fruit of a tree to a pregnant woman to induce abundance in the tree over future years. Among the Baganda people of Uganda a childless woman may be divorced because she is thought to infect her husband's garden with her own sterility. (The husband is never himself suspected.) And among the Indians of the Orinoco it is the women, not the men, who sow the fields, and with infants at the breast, in the belief that women know how to propagate most abundantly. .

Such imitative magic was often taken to greater lengths. In the ancient Greek harvest festival of Thargelia a marriage ceremony was conducted between two sacrificial victims to assist the fertilization of fig trees – a critical source of winter food. In other cultures the magic was applied in reverse: genitals would be beaten with fig branches to enhance their generative powers.

Somewhat more attractive beliefs and customs survive. In Bohemia the woman who binds the last sheaf will have a child the next year – not a fate that all necessarily would wish. In parts of Poland the last sheaf-binder is herself wrapped in the sheaf, carried home on the last wagon, drenched with water by the whole family and called 'Baba' ('Mother') until the next harvest. In parts of Bulgaria the last sheaf, often called 'the Queen', is burned and the ashes strewn on the fields to promote the fertility of the soil. And in England the Harvest Queen was often processed round the village in a carriage.

Many of the myths, rituals and monuments of different countries emphasize virility – few more than the massively equipped Cerne Abbas Giant, carved 180 feet long into the Dorset chalk. In India virgins have been cruelly deflowered with a stone lingam or phallus attributed to the god Shiva. Elsewhere the reproductive organs of animals have been scattered across the fields. The mummers' horn dance of Abbots Bromley in Staffordshire may well derive from a fertility ritual, as do the many Morris dances performed throughout the country. So, certainly, does kissing under the mistletoe, whose berries produce a liquid resembling seminal fluid.

People believe, or half believe in an extraordinary array of potions, foods, rituals and other practices with which to answer a call that goes back to Genesis (1:28): 'Be fruitful, and multiply.' Some foods are thought to induce twins. When working in South Korea, Elizabeth was told that eating a double banana would do so. Among some African tribes twins are feared, so women may be threatened with them in a curse, by way of punishment for misconduct.

Twins themselves are often believed to induce fertility and in Wales were invited to weddings for this reason. On the other hand we have met parents who groundlessly worry that one of their identical twin daughters is bound to be infertile. Parents of boy–girl pairs also worry about the daughter's fertility, wrongly believing that human twins follow the pattern of 'freemartin' calves. There, however, the female's sterility is induced by male hormones crossing the placenta from the male calf. Fortunately human boy–girl twins do not share a placenta, so the problem never arises.

Prayers for the gift of a child at particular shrines are still common although their religious connection is not always plain. While we were in Pakistan in 1992, barren women were praying at the shrine of the executed former prime minister, Zulfikar Ali Bhutto. Such practices may seem quite irrational, but the placebo effect can sometimes work.

Common Fallacies

Dubious ideas and practices also remain current in Western countries, many of them the product of historical prejudice, not least sexism. Unfortunately some of them have a superficial plausibility which may make them seriously misleading.

The false notion that infertility is essentially a woman's problem is especially prevalent. A woman's reproductive machinery is more complex than a man's, so more can go wrong, and in more obvious ways. It is the woman who either produces the child or does not. Yet about a third of all cases of infertility are due to problems in the man, and quite a lot more to a combination of problems in both partners.

Another surprisingly common fallacy is that infertility is insoluble; couples by the tens of thousand are happily disproving this. Much of the pessimism would be dispelled if couples would discuss it more openly. Infertility is neither uncommon, nor a cause for shame. True, much of it once resulted from clumsy back-street abortions, but since legalization this has become rare. Nor is infertility causally connected with a lack of femininity or masculinity. A man's 'virility' is largely irrelevant, provided he can achieve penetration and has sufficiently motile sperm. Nor does his capacity to inseminate depend on how easily or frequently he can achieve erection or orgasm, let alone on how 'manly' he appears to be, or feels.

Similarly misleading is the notion that failure to achieve pregnancy is a punishment for youthful 'misdeeds', whether masturbation, homosexual episodes or promiscuity. (Sexually transmitted diseases can, of course, have unfortunate results but may derive from just one unguarded encounter.)

Another fallacy is the suggestion that couples fail to conceive because they are of the wrong temperament or psychological combination, or have so-called character faults. For the infertile to be accused of demonstrating coldness or selfishness is both cruel and absurd.

Where couples are said to be too depressed to conceive, the chances are that the depression was caused by the infertility, not the other way round. Some infertility is certainly due to sexual or psycho-sexual difficulties, but only a very small proportion.

There are many common but false beliefs about the relationship between love-making and conception. Some couples seem to believe that the more (or less) often they make love, the more likely they are to succeed. Some think they should make love standing up or always lie down for half an hour afterwards. In Hollywood frustrated couples are said to be taking to 'organic' beds. Some couples have become so mechanical- or chart-minded in their approach that the man, especially, has been turned off intercourse altogether. Others stick rigorously to a timing formula that may have become too rigid. It is not unknown for couples systematically to miss the most favourable days!

Why Do We Want Children?

Before coming to our first overview of the latest and much more dependable methods of treating infertility, we must ask why most (though not, of course, all) of us want children in the first place.

This may not seem the most apposite question to pose to infertile couples, but there are many reasons why they particularly should consider it – if necessary with the help of a friend or a professional counsellor.

One reason is that the quest for a successful pregnancy is often long, stressful and costly in terms of time, effort and money spent. It is clearly wise for each partner to think about his or her motives before making these sacrifices. These motives will be different in kind and strength. The stability, even the survival, of the partnership may come to depend on their clarification before the almost inevitable frustrations and tensions arise.

Another reason is that any couple must be prepared for possible failure as well as success. Either will present new emotional challenges and the couple need to be as realistic as possible from the outset. Furthermore, medical staff have to assess the couple's personal suitability for treatment. Their paramount concern is bound to be the welfare of a resulting child. That must include the stability of the partnership and hence, to some degree, the degree of self-awareness of each partner and the capacity to share each other's thoughts and feelings.

Few medical professionals want to play God, and they recognize that the couple's motives are largely their own affair. But motives that are plainly poor, reckless or even frivolous are not uncommon and these may seriously affect the outlook for the would-be child. Someone who mainly wants a child in order to save a marriage should plainly wait until the situation is resolved, as should someone who is emotionally disturbed or actually mentally ill.

There are dozens of reasons why people want children. Each of us may have our own mixture of motives partly conscious, partly not.

I may want children in order to celebrate my happy partnership and literally to embody it in the form of offspring in whom our flesh, our genes and our different natures are combined. I may want children in order to give them the love I never received in childhood myself, or out of gratitude for the love I did receive. I may want to relive my own childhood or use my children to make me feel more adult.

I may seek some of the deep satisfactions of caring and being cared for that my marriage has failed to deliver. I may want to pour out my love upon my children or have them pour out their love on me.

I may want children in order to please my parents or the wider family, or to continue my family's particular bloodline. I may want them to inherit my title, my wealth, my talents or my amazing good looks. I may want them only in order to please my partner or even to stop him or her leaving me. I may not really want children at all but believe that my wider family, social circle or marriage itself somehow demands them. The longings of would-be grandparents can be especially hard to ignore.

I may, of course, want a family primarily because my religious code or my ethnic or cultural community requires it.

Or because I think it is what Nation or Nature demands. I may want children because I love the idea of children, the reality of childhood or because I want to witness and enjoy every single stage of their development from the womb, through infancy to adolescence. I may want children simply because I love children in general or because I feel a vocation for parenthood.

I may simply ache for children or weep at the thought of not having them. I may want children beyond or above or beneath any reason at all. Did I need a reason to want love, to fall in love, to want my partner? Do I need a reason to want my partner's children? Or just my own? Do any of us really need a rationalization for fulfilling what, for a majority, is so fundamental and instinctual an aspect of life? Is that not why the infertile sometimes speak of a bodily ache, a blind craving, or a want beyond tears? And why the Old Testament (Proverbs 30:16) compares a barren womb to a fire?

I, or my partner, may not want all that children may bring. Many of us could do without the inevitable strains, fears, costs, noises, smells, distractions, conflicts and disappointments. We do not need to see only the advantages.

For many couples whose pregnancies are unplanned, the children are on their way, or have even arrived, before they have thought about these issues. Others just assume that having a family is an automatic part of marriage and will not explore their motives.

Those of us who do will recognize that some of our motives may be shameful, even disgraceful. Vanity, selfishness, competitiveness, appeasement, pride, obstinacy may play a part. Some would-be parents are driven to compete with sisters or brothers, some just to rebut allegations that they are childless out of selfishness.

That particular allegation can distress not only the infertile but those who just want to remain child-free and see no reason to pretend otherwise. Women especially are too often persuaded that they cannot fulfil themselves without experiencing

29

pregnancy and motherhood. The maternal urge is not universal and in a crowded earth this is just as well. Some people do not feel 'whole' without children, others without an uninterrupted career or, indeed, solitude. Too many couples have families either by accident or to avoid appearing self-absorbed, eccentric or handicapped.

It may be as selfish for some people to have children as for others not to. Whether the abstainers are devoted to duty, money, prayer or pleasure is their business not ours.

Some of us, of course, will have neither a great longing for children nor any particular aversion to them. Many men are 'don't-knows' who are prepared to take parenthood on trust. An *Esquire* survey conducted in 1993 reported that men's most common reason was that 'their wife or partner wanted it'. One man told us how his wife had made all the running, amid great difficulties over a long period, and he had patiently gone along with it for her sake alone. But, when a baby finally arrived, he had been amazed how enthusiastic he became as soon as he took the infant to him. Then he ached for more.

Society in general puts a high value on parenting, and this can intensify the sense of inferiority, exclusion, even stigmatization, felt by the infertile. Being uncertain about one's motives is no crime, but it is especially worth trying to analyse them if, for example, one is already having some difficulties with one's partner, family or wider circle. A few partners, however, may be reluctant to discuss the subject, in the hope that it will just go away.

The Right to Have a Child?

The sheer pain of an unfulfilled longing for parenthood makes it seem brutal to pose this question, yet the more complex their motives, the more careful a couple may need to be in imposing apparently limitless demands on each other, on relatives and employers, on medical staff and perhaps taxpayers. If we have a 'right' to have a child, does this mean that no one and nothing should stand in our way? All too many of us are capable of a remorseless willingness not only to make sacrifices but to demand sacrifices of others! And for how long should we risk damaging ourselves, at least mentally, if we obsessively persist? The question of what rights we have is an issue that may be raised by medical staff and certainly by critical friends, perhaps reacting to the latest sensational article in the press.

We plainly have a moral (and legal) right not to be prevented from having a child by the arbitrary actions of others. We also have a right to receive medical advice. But to be given free treatment too, and at whose cost? What priority should be given to treating infertility compared with other medical conditions? And to whom should such treatment be made available? We shall be examining these questions later, but first let us look at the treatments currently available.

Infertility: Cure or Circumvention?

Much that is called infertility is really subfertility and, as we shall see, is now far from an absolute bar to achieving a successful pregnancy. In some cases, whether in a woman or a man, infertility is complete but may be due to causes that can be removed or cured by relatively straightforward surgery or by treatment with drugs.

On the other hand, some kinds of infertility are either essentially incurable – where, say, the ovaries or testicles have had to be removed – or would be so difficult or dangerous to remedy that a radically different strategy has to be adopted if the couple are to produce a child. In such cases the infertility must be circumvented rather than cured. Thus people who are and *remain* technically infertile become able to have children. The best-known method of achieving this is via in vitro fertilization (IVF) – that is, the 'test-tube' method. But there are other alternatives, including the donation of eggs or sperm, the use of a surrogate mother, and gamete intra-fallopian transfer (GIFT) – to which we will come shortly.

The New Reproductive Technologies: A First Overview

Some couples of whom one or other partner is to some degree subfertile can occasionally achieve a pregnancy by changing their lifestyle, but many will do so by obtaining treatment for what turns out to be either a general medical condition or a specific reproductive disorder. All that may be needed is the surgical repair to a man's vas deferens or a woman's fallopian tube. Many of these treatments are straightforward and wholly uncontroversial. So also is advice concerning psycho-sexual problems or the most favourable timing or frequency of intercourse. The use of hormone drugs to assist ovulation is another important means of remedying difficulties in conceiving and is not generally thought problematic, provided – an essential condition – that such drugs are administered in a scrupulously disciplined and monitored fashion.

Controversy did erupt, though, when it was learned how eggs could be mechanically removed from a woman's body and conception achieved by manipulation in a laboratory dish before introducing the resulting embryo into her womb. Few newspaper readers of the time will forget how, on 25 July 1978, a baby girl weighing 5 lb 12 oz, was born in Oldham General Hospital in the North of England to a worldwide fanfare of excited publicity. Her birth made history: Louise Brown was the first baby to have been conceived outside her mother's womb.

During the 1960s the scientist Robert Edwards had pioneered the fertilization of eggs outside the bodies of mice and rabbits in laboratory dishes, or 'in vitro' – literally, 'in glass'. Some of the mouse and rabbit embryos arising from these experiments were transferred into the female animals and a number of normal pregnancies and healthy offspring resulted.

Then in 1968 Bob Edwards joined Patrick Steptoe, a gynae-cologist working in Oldham. Together they researched the fertilization of human eggs and developed their techniques of in vitro fertilization and embryo transfer. By 1971 Edwards was successfully growing human embryos to the blastocyst stage (four or five days after fertilization). They reported the first human 'assisted' pregnancy in 1976 but this did not result in a live birth because the embryo became implanted in the fallopian tube. They had, however, proved it was possible to achieve a viable pregnancy, and it would only be time before a healthy baby arrived. Since the birth of Louise Brown, many other techniques of assisted conception have been developed. The three main ones are as follows:

1. In vitro fertilization (IVF) involves taking one or more eggs from the body and mixing these with sperm in a laboratory dish. When the egg is fertilized, the resultant early embryo (or embryos) is transferred to the uterus.

2. Gamete intra-fallopian transfer (GIFT) is a procedure whereby the sperm and one or more eggs are loaded into the same catheter and together transferred directly into the fal-lopian tubes to allow fertilization to occur naturally.

3. Micro-assisted fertilization (MAF) is similar to IVF but involves the use of special methods to assist the sperm in penetrating the egg in the dish before the resulting embryo is transferred to the uterus.

There are a number of other forms of assisted conception, but all are modifications of one of these three main techniques.

Two of the other new modes of treatment that circumvent infertility are not considered to provide 'assisted' conception as such. The first of these is artificial insemination (DI). Here sperm from a (usually anonymous) donor is introduced into the (fertile) woman's vagina by means of a syringe instead of by normal sexual intercourse. The other mode of treatment, surrogacy, is really one of substitute pregnancy. In this case another woman, often using the couple's eggs, sperm or embryos, agrees to carry a baby, which she intends to hand over to the couple at birth.

New Moral Dilemmas

Whereas there is little criticism of most forms of surgical and medical treatment of infertility as such, like the unblocking of fallopian tubes or the treatment of endometriosis, there has been, from the outset, fervent debate about donor insemination, surrogacy and all forms of assisted conception.

It is no wonder that such radical departures from the familiar means of conceiving, or carrying, a child should have caused such intense controversy. Almost everyone will have some concern about techniques involving the manipulation of human sperm and eggs in the laboratory, let alone the use of 'selected' donors for them.

A few may see no problems at all in using such techniques. But it should always be remembered that any damage caused to genetic material could at least theoretically affect not only the child but its own descendants for many generations to come. Indeed the very idea of assisted conception can affront our sense both of what is 'natural' and of what constitutes the 'mystery' of life. Such control over the creation of human life can seem to many a breach of sacred trust, a flouting of taboos and an act of impiety – or at least recklessness – that could have unfortunate consequences. Where, after all, might the laboratory selection of sperm, eggs and embryos lead us in a world where human ambition and greed seem limitless and all power is liable to be abused?

Aside from such weighty issues, close attention needs to be

paid to the short- and long-term implications for all involved, whether would-be parents, possible donors or surrogate mothers, medical staff and, most of all, the resulting children. Careful consideration is needed when deciding what categories of people should or should not be refused treatment or at least some kinds of it. (Some suggest lesbian or post-menopausal women should be excluded by medical ethical committees or even by law.) Who, if anyone, should get their treatment free? And what about the possible consequences of the reproductive revolution upon society as a whole, and indeed upon the size of the world population?

These complex issues will be treated in greater depth later in the book, after we have considered the nature of infertility and its investigation and treatment. But infertile couples as well as general readers may appreciate an immediate summary of the objections raised against assisted conception in particular. Couples hoping for treatment are frequently worried – even challenged by others – about this potentially painful and inflammatory subject. They may welcome forewarning about the commonest forms of criticism, without having to suffer what we would see as usually needless discouragement.

Leaders of some religious denominations argue that IVF and equivalent treatments involve a totally unacceptable 'meddling with human souls', whether through 'killing' (rejecting) some embryos or 'manufacturing' (implanting) them. Some people of entirely agnostic persuasion contend that the procedures involve an arrogant interference with natural processes or create dangerous new powers that could come to be abused by medical commerce, authoritarian governments or both. Some see so profound an intervention in the very origins of life as a kind of hubris: the reckless pride that comes before the fall. And others argue that humanity is in danger of bringing about not just procreation without coition ('babies without sex') but the separation of genetic parenthood from social parenting through the use of gamete donors.

There have been concerns about the increasing 'medicaliza-tion' of natural processes (including birth itself), about the commercialization of health care and the role of personal wealth in determining who gets what help. This is not just a worry about social justice but about the threatened 'commodifi-cation' of reproduction, whereby the child becomes just another 'thing' to be purchased or 'consumed' or where a womb could be advertised for rent. In such ways some suggest that society could be corrupted at the most basic spiritual level.

Some indeed are asking whether we are on the threshold of 'designer sperm' and 'designer ova' to produce the perfect customized baby as if selected from a catalogue. Could genetic selection and fetal diagnosis become branches of Quality Control in a state-of-the-art Child Factory where surrogate women produce pre-designed babies to order? What are the limits? Could we even be on the threshold of a eugenically controlled Brave New World run by tyrants in white coats?

A central moral – and practical – issue must be whether there will be harmful psychological effects on the resulting children. There are also fundamental questions not only about whether these treatments should be available free but whether preventive, including environmental, measures to reduce the general incidence of infertility should not have higher priority.

In Defence of Assisted Conception

As already stated, full discussion of these contentious issues comes later in the book, but having related so many objections to assisted conception, we should summarize the much more positive view taken by many others, including ourselves.

Defenders of assisted conception say that many, perhaps most, of the objections are either exaggerated or hypothetical, and that others may be overcome by a combination of profes-sional discipline and the statutory control and active monitoring of infertility clinics. They fully recognize that all new technologies entail new risks of abuse, and that neither the emotional hunger of would-be parents nor the excitement of infertility researchers should wholly determine the pace of development. But nor should the possibilities of abuse: such hypothetical dangers must always be weighed against the clear benefits to the infertile.

The new technologies have already brought about the conception and birth of treasured babies to tens of thousands of previously childless couples all over the world. They also promise to enable doctors to cure many otherwise intractable genetic diseases and to circumvent cruel genetic disabilities in generations to come.

Consideration of such benefits would not sway those who unconditionally condemn artificial conception on the grounds that the embryo has exactly the same rights as a baby and that the new procedures involve the selection and hence rejection and 'killing' of some embryos. This absolutist stance, maintained by the Vatican among other authorities, is of a piece with the condemnation of artificial birth control and abortion. Many Catholics reject the Vatican's position on all these subjects, but we consider the view of religious 'conservatives' in Chapter 12.

Professor the Reverend G. R. Dunstan made some necessary corrective observations on the subject when he opened a conference on ethics in reproductive medicine at Leeds in April 1988. He said there was almost bound to be, in Parliament and elsewhere, a restrictive mood to the effect of: 'How far can we let scientists and doctors go, and how far will they go if we do not stop them?' But disciplined curiosity, he said, was proper to the human mind and the application of knowledge to beneficial use was a duty. There was nothing noble in saying knowledge was potentially dangerous and should be brought to a standstill. Innovative medicine was a proper duty and high vocation for the human mind. And for Christians, he said –

speaking as an ordained priest – it was proper work for man made in the image of God.[1]

It is plainly right that there should be a wide-ranging public debate of both the general principles in question and of the balance of dangers and benefits. Most of the infertile will welcome most of the emerging techniques, provided these are carefully regulated and sensitively applied. What this means in practice will be discussed in the chapters that follow.

3. Normal Procreation

To understand infertility we must first understand fertility. For five women out of six, getting pregnant appears to be so easy that they have no need to think about it – except sometimes with apprehension: some find pregnancy hard to avoid. In the UK, for instance, about one-third of pregnancies are unplanned and a substantial proportion of these are actually unwanted.

Technically speaking, fertility is defined as the number of babies actually produced, whereas the capacity of women to produce children, whether they do or not, is termed fecundity. This potentially confusing nomenclature need not, however, detain us for long. The general 'fertility' rate in any given population is defined as the number of liveborn children delivered annually per thousand women of between fifteen and forty-four years of age, a rate that varies over time. Taking the UK over the last fifty years, the rate peaked in 1964, at 93 per thousand, and then fell until 1977, when it was 58. There has since been a slight upward trend: 64 per thousand in 1990, for instance.

The mean maternal age at childbirth in Britain has risen over recent years, from 26.2 years in 1974 to 28.7 in 1990. Women are also tending to have their first child later, at an average age of twenty-eight years in 1992 compared with twenty-four in 1965. An increasing number of women are waiting until their late thirties or even early forties before trying to start a family. Recent figures show that for the first time more women in their thirties are becoming pregnant than in their twenties.

In many countries families are becoming smaller. The current average number of children in a British family is, by European standards, quite high. Since the late 1980s Britain's fertility rate – the average number of children born per woman of child-bearing age – has been 1.9. In some countries, like Germany, and even, contrary to expectation, Spain and Italy, the figures are lower, at 1.5, 1.4 and 1.3 respectively. This is below the level needed to sustain their present populations.

An increasing number of children are being born outside marriage. In the UK the percentage has risen from 5 per cent in 1960 to 28 per cent in 1990. Nevertheless many of these children are born into stable relationships, unmarried but committed (and many of the parents marry later), so hasty judgements about this phenomenon may well prove facile if not simply false.

A woman has the potential to become pregnant throughout the period of her life that her ovaries are releasing eggs. In most women ovulation starts a few months after the first menstrual period. The average age for the onset of menstruation is thirteen years, with the great majority of girls starting between the ages of eleven and fifteen, and continues until the menopause, which normally occurs at about fifty years of age.

There are rare examples of pregnancies in very young children, but this only occurs where there is a disorder causing some form of hormonal imbalance, accompanied, of course, by impregnation. There have also been examples of especially elderly motherhood. The oldest woman reliably known to have had a naturally conceived live birth was a Californian who had a daughter at the age of fifty-seven years and 129 days.

There are many trials and obstacles to be overcome between the production of a single egg, achieving a pregnancy and the arrival of a baby. In any one month the average chance of achieving a pregnancy lies between 15 and 25 per cent. Women aged between twenty and twenty-five have the best chance of conception. After the mid-thirties a woman's fertility declines rapidly. At thirty-five the average time taken to get pregnant is six months, whereas at twenty-five it is two to three months.

The process of procreation is so complex that one wonders that so many women do get pregnant, not that some have problems. We shall look at the four essential ingredients for procreation in turn: the egg, the sperm, an opportunity for them to meet at the right time, and a safe environment in which the united egg and sperm can develop. (Readers who know the physiology well may wish to pass straight on to the next chapter.)

The Egg

Human eggs – ova or oocytes – are produced by the two ovaries which lie either side of the lower part of the female abdomen. By the fifth month of pregnancy the female fetus has ovaries containing some seven million eggs. This number has already fallen to two million by birth and to 400,000 by puberty. However, there are plenty to spare since most women use only about 350 eggs in their 30–40 years of potentially reproductive life.

Various hormones are essential to the stages of development, from the rudimentary ovum to the mature single egg that is shed in the middle of the normal menstrual cycle. A region in the lower part of the brain, called the hypothalamus, regulates the pituitary gland – a pea-sized structure situated at the base of the skull. This gland produces the hormones which influence the action of other glands in various parts of the body, including the ovaries and the testicles. An ovary responds by maturing an egg and the testicles by producing sperm.

At the beginning of the menstrual cycle the hypothalamus signals the pituitary gland to release a follicle-stimulating hormone (FSH), which stimulates a number of follicles in the ovary. Over the next two weeks twenty or so follicles develop, each containing an egg. While they do so they produce oestrogen, a hormone which enters the bloodstream and tells the pituitary gland to reduce the amount of FSH, thereby limiting its effect to only one follicle in the ovary. The remaining follicles shrivel up.

Secondly the oestrogen stimulates the pituitary to produce another hormone – luteinizing hormone (LH). LH and FSH are together known as the gonadotrophins. In a normal 28-day cycle a surge of LH occurs after twelve days and this causes the follicle to ripen. Then, 28–32 hours later, ovulation takes place, with the release of the mature egg into the abdomen just near the entrance – the ampulla – to one of the two fallopian tubes which lead to the womb.

The Sperm

The production of sperm – or spermatozoa – is a continuous process and the 'normally' fertile man is fertile every day from puberty to a relatively late age, in marked contrast to the woman, who is fertile for only a few days each month. In old age many men can produce sperm but not many are fertile. We should remember that maternity is a question of fact whereas paternity is usually a matter of assumption. (It has been suggested that about 10 per cent of the population may not have been sired by the man they believe to be their father.)

Sperm are formed in the seminiferous tubules in the testes. These coils of tubes lead into a larger tube, the epididymis, also coiled, which in turn leads into a single large tube, the vas deferens. Sperm production (and maturation) is stimulated by the same pituitary hormones, FSH and LH, as are produced in the woman. FSH stimulates the seminiferous tubules to produce sperm. LH stimulates specialized cells, the Leydig cells, to secrete the hormone testosterone, which is responsible for the development of male physical characteristics as well as enhancing the production of sperm. FSH and testosterone stimulate the immature sperm to develop into mature sperm.

Each sperm has a head which contains the genetic material, a neck which enables it to swim and a tail which propels it through the female genital tract. A sperm is about 0.05 mm long, or approximately one-500th of an inch. Unlike the woman, who is born with her full complement of eggs, the male is continuously producing sperm from puberty onwards.

Sperm take about sixty days to mature and another two weeks or so to pass along the coils of tubes to the vas deferens. Here they wait for the next male orgasm, when they will be ejaculated in the semen. In addition to sperm, semen contains fluid from the seminal vesicles and glands, including the prostate, which provides nourishment, as well as a vehicle, for the sperm.

About 200–300 million sperm are ejaculated into the vagina, but only 100–200 actually make contact with an egg. Most are either lost by trickling out of the vagina or by swimming into the abdominal cavity from the fallopian tubes. Others are destroyed by the natural acidity of the vagina, if they do not pass through to the alkaline environment of the uterus quickly enough. Even if they make it to the uterus, some will be destroyed by endometrial cells lining the womb. Moreover the condition of the mucus of the cervix (the neck of the womb) is only suitable for the passage of the sperm for a few days during the monthly cycle.

Fertilization

After the egg has been released from the ovary, fimbria (the very fine, finger-like processes at the opening to the fallopian tubes) waft the egg into the opening or ampulla of the fallopian tube, and it is here that fertilization takes place.

Clearly the sperm must reach the ampulla at the right time.

Although some will reach it within a few minutes of intercourse, others will be stored in reservoirs in the mucus of the
cervix, from where they are released at intervals into the
uterine cavity. A sperm can survive and remain active for two
to four days and occasionally up to seven. Therefore, although
the egg is only fertilizable for about twenty-four hours, there
is some leeway in the timing of intercourse.

After ovulation the empty follicle forms what is known
as the corpus luteum, which itself produces another hormone,
progesterone. This, together with oestrogen, acts on the lining
of the womb, the endometrium, to prepare it to receive the
egg, should it be fertilized. If the egg is not fertilized, the
level of progesterone gradually falls, the endometrium sheds
its lining and a new menstrual period will start approximately fourteen days after ovulation. Then the cycle begins
again.

The egg does not appear to have a particular means of
attracting a sperm to it, so it is chance whether they meet.
Luckily there are usually so many sperm that the chances are
quite good. Around the egg is a capsule, the zona pellucida,
which allows only one sperm to penetrate it and then
promptly forms an impenetrable barrier to all other
candidates.

After it has penetrated the egg, the head of the fertilizing
sperm releases its contents which move towards the nucleus of
the egg. Fertilization then takes place and the egg divides first
into two cells, then four, eight, sixteen and so on. Over the
next thirty hours the newly developing embryo travels down
the fallopian tube to the uterus.

In the four days following fertilization the embryo develops
into a solid ball of cells, the morula. This enlarges, absorbs
fluid and becomes a blastocyst – a single layer of cells surrounding the fluid. Approximately five days after ovulation this
enters the uterus and becomes embedded in the endometrium.
The endometrium responds by producing a hormone called

human chorionic gonadotrophin (HCG) and all pregnancy tests are based on the detection of this hormone either in the blood or the urine.

4. The Nature of Infertility, and its Investigation

Some couples seem to assume that, once they have decided to have a baby, it will duly arrive nine months later – like ordering the groceries for Friday. But even a young, normally fertile woman, having regular sexual intercourse with a normally fertile partner, will have only a one-in-four chance of becoming pregnant in any given month. In women over thirty the chances get smaller. The overall average time taken to become pregnant is six months.

It is clear, therefore, that many couples start feeling anxious long before they need to. When *should* a couple begin to worry? The usual definition of infertility is a failure to conceive within one year of regular, unprotected sexual intercourse. Two years might be a more appropriate criterion since many couples will conceive during the second year without treatment. However, the older you are, the earlier you probably need to seek help. (Going on to a waiting list for treatment is often said to be one of the most effective ways of achieving conception!)

There have been cases of couples conceiving spontaneously after many years of unprotected intercourse, long after they had abandoned any hopes of parenthood, let alone plans for it. In general, though, the chance of pregnancy falls substantially if you have not conceived after two years of unprotected intercourse.

True infertility is a total inability to conceive without medical intervention. This is relatively uncommon, so in most cases the more accurate term would be subfertility. However, as infertility is now the term generally applied to anyone having difficulty in becoming pregnant, we too will mostly use this expression.

A full understanding of infertility by the medical profession is a long way off, but there are various extreme points of view, each of which, taken alone, seems inadequate or worse. One such viewpoint, obviously false, is that infertility is the result of some sort of curse that the victim must just accept. Simple observation of the very many couples who conceive after treatment dismisses such fatalism.

Some see infertility as essentially a spiritual or moral matter for which only prayer or spiritual healing can provide an answer. Others say that it is a question of psychology, essentially remediable only by some form of psychotherapy. Another approach argues that infertility can be wholly accounted for in bodily or physiological terms and can only be dealt with by drugs, surgery or technical 'fixes' like IVF.

All three of these perspectives – spiritual, psychological and physical – probably have some value and should perhaps be combined in a single holistic view. There will be some cases where attention to just one aspect – say, a surgical unblocking – can remedy the situation. More often, however, couples will do best to bear in mind all three perspectives. This is especially worth remembering when we describe each treatment separately, as if it were only a technical procedure.

The exact prevalence of infertility is difficult to establish, partly because many people never reveal, or even recognize, their disability. The number of involuntarily childless women, and indeed couples, is therefore unknown. Unfortunately many frustrated people never seek help, so cannot take advantage of the services that are available. In some parts of the UK fewer than half of those believed to be having difficulty actually seek medical advice. Even so, estimates can still be made, and on current evidence about one in six couples appear to have some difficulty in conceiving.

A Canadian study showed that 8.5 per cent of couples, who had been married or cohabiting for at least a year (and did not use contraception), failed to get pregnant. On this basis there would be over a quarter of a million Canadian couples experiencing infertility, and about double that number of British couples similarly afflicted. Currently three women in twenty in the UK remain childless but the figure is rising. The Office of Population, Censuses and Surveys estimates that one in five women born in 1980 will not have children. But then many of these will have chosen not to.

Infertility can be divided into two categories: primary and secondary. Primary infertility is never having achieved a pregnancy. Secondary infertility is where the couple is currently having difficulty but has had at least one pregnancy together. Each category makes up about half the total number of infertile.

There are also cases of couples where each member has had a successful pregnancy with previous partners, but who are not managing to have a child together. Sometimes this is because either or both have had an infection since the last pregnancy, but often there is no discovered cause.

In both primary and secondary groups about half of the cases will be remediable and, sooner or later, they will have a child. In the end 3–4 per cent of those couples who are actively trying to have a child will fail ever to have one of their own, even if they are lucky enough to have access to all current forms of treatment.

Since the 1970s there appears to have been some increase in the numbers of involuntarily childless couples. As we will discuss shortly, a decline in male fertility has been suspected in recent decades. The current trend towards a later age of childbearing is also likely to result in more couples being childless because of the fall in the woman's fertility after the age of thirty. Many women are now continuing longer with their education or training and are more committed to their career. Others want to create a secure – or even a fully equipped – home before starting a family.

For those who wait until their late thirties there is less time for the protracted process of recognizing first that there is a problem, then of joining a waiting list for investigation, then another for one treatment, and perhaps others for a second or third. Time can run out.

Seeking Help

It is not easy to say when a couple should seek help. Some couples fear something is wrong if the female partner is not pregnant two weeks after their first attempt. Others go on trying for years, quietly assuming a baby will arrive in its own good time. In effect some couples seek advice months before they need to and some wait years longer than they should. There is certainly no need to ask for help within the first six months unless there are any of the untoward signs discussed later in this chapter. Beyond six months couples should seek advice as soon as they feel worried.

After six months couples still have a very good chance of conceiving spontaneously, and where the woman has not reached her late thirties, little is lost in waiting at least for another six months to see what happens. For those over thirty-five it is probably sensible to seek help earlier.

For most people the easiest and most appropriate person to see first is their family doctor. Those who are hesitant about this, for whatever reason, can contact one of the self-help organizations such as ISSUE (formerly the National Association for the Childless), who will gladly give all sorts of information and advice (see Where to Find Help for the address). Not only will they encourage a couple to seek a medical opinion but they will help them prepare for the questions that will be asked.

After hearing the couple's story, the doctor will usually offer some useful suggestions and say whether they should wait a while or undergo preliminary investigations. Most family doctors will undertake some of these themselves, whether of the woman, the man or both. Others will refer their patients straight to a specialist. This will largely depend on their own experience and the philosophy of the local infertility clinic.

The general practitioner and the specialist will always prefer to see both partners. But what if one member of the couple refuses to acknowledge the problem or to seek help? There is no reason why one partner should not go on his or her own, although this too may create tensions between them both. However, the doctor may be able to advise the willing partner how to understand and perhaps overcome the reluctance of the other. Time and patience may be needed. Counsellors from ISSUE are well used to helping in such situations.

Usually, but not always, the reluctance is greatest in the male partner. Quite irrationally, some men feel subfertility would be a slight on their virility or manhood. This is nonsense. Nevertheless we have encountered several cases where the male partner has refused to discuss the possibility of a semen analysis, either with his partner or his doctor. (The 'refuser' may sometimes be persuaded to change his mind by getting him to read a relevant article or book.)

The reluctant male should be made to realize that many women have undergone painful and often unnecessary tests because their partner has declined to have one or two simple and painless ones himself. Nowadays most specialists would not continue investigations of the woman until a semen specimen had been analysed. It is both unkind to the woman and potentially wasteful of everyone's time and effort.

The doctor will first take a careful history of both partners' general health, and then of the woman's menstrual cycle, previous pregnancies (if any) and past infections. He or she will also probably ask the couple about their sexual behaviour: the timing and frequency of intercourse and any problems there may be.

Clearly the mechanics must be right. The doctor will examine the woman to check the health of the vagina and cervix, and will feel for any enlargement or tenderness of the womb, fallopian tubes or ovaries. The man's testes will be examined for their size and for any problems such as varicoceles (discussed later). Abnormalities of the penis that might interfere with insemination, such as a hypospadias (incomplete development of the penis), will also be looked for.

Occasionally the egg and sperm fail to meet because intercourse is incomplete or otherwise unsatisfactory. Sometimes this is due to a mechanical difficulty such as an imperforate hymen – the membrane at the entrance of the vagina that is normally broken by intercourse – which prevents penetration. This can usually be corrected by stretching the membrane, but occasionally the obstruction is more substantial and minor plastic surgery is called for.

In other cases penetration may be prevented by vaginismus – a spasm in the muscles of the vaginal wall which narrows the entrance to the vagina. This distressing condition may occur whenever intercourse is attempted. To overcome it, psycho-sexual counselling may be required, usually involving both partners. Sometimes this takes a while to achieve success.

If the preliminary investigations reveal no problems, some screening tests will probably be carried out to check whether the man is producing enough active sperm and whether the female partner is ovulating regularly. There may, of course, be a number of contributory factors even if one problem dominates, and this should be borne in mind when reading the next section where the problems are set out separately.

Some couples might have had little difficulty in conceiving if the problem lay with one partner. A combination of factors on both sides can tilt the balance. For instance, a somewhat low sperm count might not have mattered if the female partner had been younger or not experiencing irregular ovulation.

The prevalence of any particular disorder in the general

population is hard to establish because the kind and number of problems dealt with in each clinic will vary partly with the population served and partly with the particular expertise or reputation of the specialists involved. (Where there is known to be an expert on a particular disorder, afflicted couples will naturally travel further and wait longer to attend that clinic.)

Male Infertility

Male infertility of various kinds and origins currently affects at least one man in twenty and is responsible for about a third of childlessness, much of it being relatively difficult to treat. Its prevalence has long been underestimated, and not least by the medical profession. Many men produce too few sperm (referred to as oligospermia), rather than none at all (azoospermia). Some produce enough sperm, but these do not move energetically enough following ejaculation. This is known as impaired motility.

Defects in the production of sperm may be due to various causes. One is poor hormone production as a result of abnormalities in the hypothalamus/pituitary function. Another is a congenital abnormality of the testes such as lack of development, or hypogonadism. Hypogonadism is often associated with undescended testes, which in turn may or may not be due to a specific syndrome, such as Klinefelter's, in which the men have an extra X (female) chromosome.

Sperm production may fail because of tumours of the testes or damage to them from radiation or from drugs or infections such as mumps. An accident to a testis may stop the blood supply to it and cause irreversible damage. So may a twisting or torsion of the testis. However, as long as the other testis remains unscathed, fertility should not be affected, as a single testis usually produces more than enough sperm with which to fertilize an egg. On the other hand, damage caused by mumps, radiation or drugs may often involve both testes.

General illness, both acute and chronic, can have remarkable effects on the quality and quantity of the sperm. Sometimes a short feverish illness, like influenza, can temporarily stop sperm production altogether. For this reason no diagnosis or conclusion should ever be reached on the strength of a single low sperm count. The test should always be repeated, usually after a month and sometimes again a month later.

Cigarette smoking decreases the number and motility of sperm, as can alcohol, although the main harm here lies in the reduction in libido. Impotence is a common side-effect of drinking excessive quantities of alcohol. There are also a number of drugs, including one commonly used in the treatment of epilepsy, which can suppress sperm production. Fortunately there are alternatives which do not do so: a family doctor would give advice on these matters.

Some men produce antibodies against their own sperm. These antibodies damage the sperm so that they clump together and lose their normal ability to swim forwards.

Abstinence from sexual intercourse is often but wrongly recommended as a means of improving sperm production. There are no grounds for believing it helps – indeed the conserved sperm may die off and the average quality of the semen may therefore deteriorate. On the other hand, very frequent ejaculations can reduce sperm counts to zero.

Sperm may be produced but not released from the testes due to an obstruction of the epididymis or the tube leading from it, the vas deferens. Such obstructions may result from a congenital abnormality or infection, from radiation or an irreversible sterilization.

An absence of the vas deferens is responsible for about one per cent of male infertility. It is a recognized and probably invariable complication of the hereditary disease cystic fibrosis (whose main symptoms are respiratory and digestive). In California Dr Pasquale Patrizio has shown that in a substantial number of men the absence of the vas deferens may be the only sign of an unusual or mild form of cystic fibrosis, which itself often remains undetected.[1] Such men would be well advised to seek genetic counselling.

The role of varicoceles – deformed and swollen veins surrounding the testis – in causing infertility is uncertain. It has been suggested that sperm production may be suppressed by the change in temperature resulting from the increased blood flow in the varicoceles.

Defects in the transport of the sperm may also be due to problems with ejaculation, including premature ejaculation and difficulty in achieving or sustaining an erection (impotence). Effective transport of the sperm requires an adequate volume of seminal fluid, and this may be reduced if the glands producing it are damaged.

Environmental Dangers

In October 1993 a BBC *Horizon* programme alerted the British people to possible threats to male fertility from pollutants in their water supplies. A Danish endocrinologist, Dr Niels Skakkebaek, had proposed at a recent Washington conference that oestrogen-mimicking pollutants may underlie what he believed to be a disturbing drop in sperm counts since the 1930s. Among nearly 15,000 men studied by the Danish Department of Growth and Reproduction, the average sperm count had fallen from 113 million per ml. in 1940 to 66 million per ml. in 1990. The volume had also dropped by about one-fifth. Moreover an increasing number of sperm showed abnormalities (such as grossly distorted or entirely absent heads) or appeared motionless or hyperactive. In addition the incidence of undescended testicles in newborn boys was said to have doubled since the 1950s (to nearly 3 per cent), and testicular cancer had reportedly trebled in fifty years. Then a study at a university hospital in Paris (*Guardian*, 15 February 1995) reported that the average sperm count of Parisian men had declined by almost a third between 1973 and 1992 and suggested the decline was continuing.

Other medical authorities have contested these findings, including their statistical validity, and the jury must be regarded as still 'out'. There are, however, serious grounds for concern, not least since the quality of 'normal' human sperm is already very poor compared with that of other mammalian species. Current American research may produce more definitive findings.

Oestrogen is produced by men as well as women. In the male it stimulates the Sertoli cells in the developing embryo to produce secretions which promote the growth of the male reproductive organs. Oestrogen imitators are said to be all around us: in many pesticides and fertilizers, for instance; in the PCBs used as coolants in older refrigerators; and the polycarbonate plastics often used in bottles. These oestrogen imitators are therefore present in the soil, lakes and rivers – and even the air – and hence possibly in our water supplies. So, some fear, are accumulating residues from contraceptive pills. Clearly this is a subject deserving urgent further study.

Investigation

As one of the initial screening tests the man will be asked to produce a specimen of semen into a jar, and this must be examined within an hour and a half of ejaculation to estimate the number of sperm, their motility and their structure.

A sperm count of 20 million per ml. is regarded as satisfactory. Conception may still occur normally when the count is much lower, provided the female partner has a normal level of fertility. Of the sperm seen in the specimen, over 40 per cent should be motile and progressive, but sperm with a much lower motility rate can be used in IVF procedures. Some sperm will be observed to have abnormal forms, but again at least 40 per cent should have a normal structure. White blood cells are also counted because an excess of these may indicate the presence of an infection.

When the couple's problem turns out to be partly or entirely on the man's side, it is often a shock to both partners. Male infertility is so rarely discussed that it is usually unexpected. Nor has the man usually had warning signs of anything being wrong. After seven years of fruitless trying and unnecessary tests on herself, one woman described her reaction: 'The news hit us like a bombshell . . . I had never considered this possibility, looking at my strapping, handsome partner.'

Many men regard their infertility, however illogically, as a threat to their virility and masculinity, and this in itself can trigger sexual problems, reinforcing the sense of failure. Impotence is not uncommon immediately after the diagnosis of male infertility and usually lasts for a few months. Men have been known to offer their wives a divorce at this time. Both partners need to exercise the utmost patience with each other.

A male infertility test kit developed in Belgium recently came on to the British market (at around £20 for a pack of two tests). Satisfactory sperm production is said to be indicated if a dye which has been mixed with the semen turns from deep purple to pink, as this only happens if enough active, oxygen consuming sperm are present. The developers hoped that, in this easy private way, more men would test themselves at an early stage and hence spare many women the distress of unnecessary testing. However, we cannot ourselves vouch for the reliability of the test.

Female Infertility

In contrast to men, women are often not at all surprised to find they are having trouble in conceiving. A woman's menstrual periods may have been erratic or scanty, suggesting a problem with ovulation. She may have had an unusual amount of pain at the time of ovulation or deep pain during intercourse. This might indicate endometriosis or adhesions due to previous infection, perhaps following a burst appendix. Such matters are likely to be the first thing the doctor will ask about before starting any specific investigations.

Female infertility can be due to problems in producing eggs (ovulation) or with their transport or with both. Problems with ovulation can be divided into those resulting from a failure in the ovaries themselves and those due to a disorder in the hormones controlling the ovaries.

Primary Ovarian Failure

This occurs if the ovaries have been removed or permanently damaged by, say, radiation treatment. In some genetic diseases, such as Turner's syndrome (where a woman has only one, instead of two, sex chromosomes), the ovaries fail to develop in the first place.

The most common reason for ovulation to stop is the menopause: the ovaries just run out of viable eggs. This does not usually occur until a woman has reached her late forties or early fifties, but premature menopause can occur in a woman's thirties or even twenties and can be a shattering experience. (Increasing numbers of women are now seeking help who have become sterile as a result of an earlier course of radiotherapy or chemotherapy treatment for cancer.) At present, once the menopause has occurred it cannot be reversed, and the only chance of a pregnancy lies through egg donation (see Chapter 6). It may in future become possible to restore ovarian function through the transplantation of ovarian tissue, though this may never become a routine procedure.

Secondary Ovarian Failure

Here the ovaries may themselves be normal but fail to release viable eggs due to a disturbance in the woman's hormonal balance. This is a highly technical subject which most readers will not need to conquer, but a summary may be useful.

Up to 60 per cent of ovulatory problems are caused by polycystic ovary disease. In this case the menstrual cycle is prolonged due to an excessive secretion of testosterone, which in turn leads to an imbalance between LH and FSH. As a result the ovaries become full of little cysts and the ovarian follicle fails to develop normally.

If insufficient FSH is produced by the pituitary gland, there will be an inadequate luteal phase and the ovarian follicle will not then be prepared to respond to the rise in LH which would normally lead to ovulation. Even if ovulation does take place, the remaining corpus luteum will be unable to produce the normal levels of progesterone to stimulate the endometrium to prepare for implantation of the embryo.

If the pituitary gland or the hypothalamus should fail to act properly, reproduction would be just one of the many body functions to suffer. The failure may be due to a developmental defect or to a tumour. Pituitary function may also diminish in times of great stress or weight loss and can be a problem for gymnasts, long-distance runners and even dancers. Removal of the stress and increase in weight will usually cure the problem without any form of hormone treatment. However it is not uncommon for menstruation to be delayed for up to a year after normal weight has been regained. Anorexia in teenage girls and young women is a not uncommon but very distressing cause of infertility and usually requires prolonged help from a psychiatrist or psychotherapist.

Reduced or absent ovulation may be caused by hyperprolacti-naemia (an increased concentration of prolactin in the blood), a condition in which excessive production of the pituitary hormone prolactin interferes with the production of FSH and LH. Hyperprolactinaemia also explains why women are unlikely to conceive while breastfeeding.

Preliminary Tests for Ovulation

The best-known test for checking ovulation is the temperature chart – produced by taking one's temperature first thing each morning and charting the readings. These should show a rise of about half a degree centigrade at the time of ovulation. Yet temperature charts can be misleading: some women experience a rise in temperature without ovulation and others ovulate normally without a rise showing on their chart. A feverish illness will, in any case, throw the record into chaos. Many specialists now favour abandoning these charts as more sophisticated tests for detecting ovulation have become available. For example, a blood test taken in the mid-luteal phase (about seven days before the expected onset of the next menstrual period) will measure the amount of progesterone present and thereby provide a good indication as to whether ovulation has taken place.

If physical examination of both partners reveals nothing wrong, the sperm is normal and the mid-luteal blood test indicates ovulation, there is a very good chance of a spontaneous pregnancy within a year or so. Some doctors would then recommend waiting for a second year unless the woman is past her middle thirties, or has some definite reason to believe something is amiss. Other practitioners feel there is no good reason for delaying at this stage.

Seeking a Specialist's Opinion

Sooner or later, if no baby has arrived, most couples will ask their doctor (or other 'primary' health adviser) for a referral to an infertility clinic either within their District Hospital's general gynaecology unit or at a specialized, so-called 'tertiary', centre. In some District Hospitals (or 'secondary' units) there will be a doctor who specializes in infertility, but more commonly one of the general gynaecologists will take a particular interest in it.

In the UK the National Health Service aims to provide a unit specializing in infertility for every half million people. (As we shall see, the number of fully specialized 'tertiary' centres is in fact a quarter of this. Their geographical distribution is also very uneven and their waiting lists are long.)

The priority given to infertility treatment in Britain varies greatly from one District Health Authority to another. Some strictly limit the range of available treatments. Some will not perform DI. Assisted conception is very difficult to obtain, even if the patient is able to make a contribution to the costs. Some Authorities provide GIFT but offer IVF only to few, if any, couples. Some seem to regard anything beyond treatment with hormones as a very low priority, even a dispensable luxury, along with the removal of tattoos or unsightly varicose veins. We will discuss these issues in more detail in Chapter 14.

Family doctors will advise about the current options available for treatment in their area, and the likely waiting times. All too many people will find themselves forced to consider private treatment, if they can afford it.

Again ISSUE can provide helpful information about the services available in different NHS areas and in private clinics, and the speed with which treatment might be expected. Shopping around is recommended in order to get information both on success rates and, where relevant, prices, which can vary considerably.

Investigating the Transport of the Eggs

If the preliminary tests have suggested that ovulation is occurring normally, the next stage is to check the transport of the eggs. Once the egg is released from the ovaries, a clear passage is obviously essential for the egg to complete its journey, which may be interrupted in a number of ways.

Blocked Fallopian Tubes

Blockages most commonly result from scarring and adhesions following inflammation in the pelvis. This can be due to irradiation or sexually transmitted infection, or occur after a burst appendix or as a result of damage from an intra-uterine contraceptive device. Infections following abortion are now rare, and many people worry unnecessarily about this.

Endometriosis

This condition also causes adhesions in the abdomen and is responsible for about 20 per cent of female infertility. It is a condition in which some of the endometrial tissue normally lining the cavity of the womb becomes detached and is re-implanted in the cavity of the abdomen. Here it will respond to hormones in the same way as the endometrium in the womb, bleeding and shedding tissue during the menstrual cycle. This tissue in the abdomen can cause inflammation and scarring which often distort the reproductive organs or block the fallopian tubes. The adhesions may prevent the ova being released from the ovaries or block their passage in the fallopian tubes.

Fibroids

Fibroids are non-malignant ('benign') tumours composed of extra amounts of the muscle and fibrous tissue making up the walls of the uterus. They may be present in great numbers and vary in size from a tiny lump to something as big as a grapefruit, or even larger. In themselves they are not harmful but their sheer size may cause infertility by obstructing a fallopian tube or by distorting the shape of the womb and hence preventing implantation.

Other Conditions

Abnormalities of the uterus such as a divided ('bicornuate') uterus may cause problems, but often they have no ill effect on either fertility or pregnancy. Normal pregnancies can occur even when the uterus is entirely divided.

Sometimes, although there may be no problem with the transport of the eggs, the sperm are unable to reach them. The mucus of the cervix normally thins in the middle of the monthly cycle. But if the mucus remains thick and sticky during the crucial mid-cycle days, when the sperm need to be able to swim quickly and easily into the uterus, the sperm may be delayed so that they die off before reaching the uterus. Furthermore the woman as well as the man may produce antibodies to sperm, and if these appear in the cervical mucus, they too may cause damage.

Next Steps

The order in which subsequent investigations are carried out will depend partly on the leads so far obtained.

If a difficulty is suspected in the pick-up and passage of the ova, an examination of the woman's reproductive organs – the ovaries, uterus and fallopian tubes – will be needed. This usually first takes the form of an abdominal or vaginal ultrasound scan to give a general view of the abdomen. An X-ray such as a hysterosalpingogram (HSG) may also be performed. This involves injecting dye into the womb through the cervix to show whether there are any abnormalities such as a blockage of one or both tubes. The test is usually carried out if a tubal blockage is suspected or if there have been recurrent miscarriages.

A laparoscopy may then follow. Here an instrument like a very small mobile telescope is inserted into the abdomen so that all the organs can be carefully examined. At the same time some dye may be injected through the cervix to see if it flows normally through the uterus and up the fallopian tubes. More recently hysteroscopy has become available, in which the 'telescope' is introduced into the womb itself so that the interior can be examined. A tiny scraping or biopsy of the endometrium may also be taken to exclude the presence of any infection and to confirm that there are signs of ovulation.

Problems of Ovulation

Further measurements of the hormone levels in the blood may indicate where the core problem lies. A high level of FSH will suggest that the ovaries are not responding normally to stimulation. Ultrasound scans may already have revealed polycystic ovaries. If there is too high a level of prolactin, this may be due to the presence of a small pituitary tumour secreting high levels of prolactin, to a shortage of thyroid hormone, to certain drugs such as phenothiazines, or sometimes, as in the case of athletes, to undue emotional or physical stress.

An X-ray of the skull to show the cavity housing the pituitary gland – the pituitary fossa – will often reveal if there is any enlargement of the gland that could result in the secretion of an abnormal amount of hormones, such as prolactin. More detailed examinations might then be needed.

Unexplained Infertility

All the test results, in both the man and woman, may turn out to be perfectly normal or at least reveal nothing sufficiently abnormal to explain the difficulty in conceiving. We ourselves were in this category and, like many others, found the lack of an explanation very frustrating. If a problem is identified, it may be treatable and at least the persistent uncertainty is removed. As many as a third of all couples attending infertility clinics can discover no explanation for their infertility, although the proportion varies with the types of patient attending any given clinic and is decreasing as more sophisticated tests become available to a larger number of couples.

If both partners appear to be normally fertile, the next tests will probably be aimed at finding out whether there is some sort of incompatibility between them. A post-coital test taken at the time of ovulation can show whether the mucus of the cervix is compatible with the sperm and whether insemination can take place. Between six and twelve hours after intercourse a specimen of mucus from the cervix is examined under the microscope. Active sperm should be visible in each view. Repeated abnormal results may be due to failure of ejaculation, inadequate production of cervical mucus or to the presence of antibodies which inhibit the sperm.

As in other rapidly advancing fields, there are many different medical opinions regarding the different types of investigation and treatment. Some specialists, for example, try IVF far sooner than others, arguing that the ability of the sperm to fertilize the egg can be tested at the same time. They say this saves unnecessary delay, anxiety and cost, compared with going through both procedures separately. Others argue that the couple should be investigated more thoroughly first, before trying IVF.

Some couples will have been referred directly to a specialist or 'tertiary' unit by their family doctor. Others will be sent to one when their District Hospital is unable to establish the cause of the infertility. Whether either will provide the necessary treatment, should this be GIFT or IVF, is another matter.

Counselling

There can be few more bewildering and stressful experiences than those encountered in an infertile couple's quest for a child. In the past most couples struggled with inadequate information, less guidance and little support during an often unforgivably long process. If finally successful, they were often left in the dark about ensuing problems, like what to tell the child. If they finally failed to have a child, they had little help in coping with their bereavement. Many couples also lacked advice in working through the problems that had almost inevitably arisen in their own relationship.

With notable exceptions the UK's counselling services for the infertile have been abysmally inadequate. The Human Fertilisation and Embryology (HFE) Act of 1990, however, insists that counselling be made available to all couples receiving treatment in a licensed centre, to all those considering donating gametes or embryos and to any children who, after the age of eighteen, wish to gain further information about their genetic origins.

At first there was inevitably a shortage of appropriately trained counsellors but now a body of them is developing, supported by such organizations as the British Infertility Counselling Association (BICA). Nevertheless some couples are still reluctant to use the service, regarding any need for counselling as some sort of weakness. (Men are especially prone to feel this yet are those most often in need of it.) Counselling should be seen as an integral and natural part of the overall therapy, available to both partners, separately and together.

How much counselling any particular couple will need, and of what emphasis, will be mainly up to them. There are said to be four main aspects to counselling: the supplying of information: the discussion of implications; the provision of support; and then, where necessary, the offering of therapy. In general couples are well advised to give each of these aspects the benefit of any initial doubt. At the very least couples find the process a valuable learning experience, often with wider benefits. We summarize each in turn.

Information Counselling

All couples should receive factual information and advice about any investigation or treatment and its likely outcome. (Some would not consider this part of counselling as such.) Information like this should be provided automatically by the specialist, but the couple may well wish to talk some of it over with a second person who has more time. Written information is essential and is usually provided by the treatment centre. Useful leaflets are also published by the Human Fertilisation and Embryology Authority (HFEA) and a number of voluntary organizations.

Implications Counselling

The couple will also need help in exploring the implications of the options open to them, both for themselves and for others concerned, including any existing child. This exploration sometimes involves potentially painful emotions and may require time and a sensitive approach. Issues that are at once very practical and highly emotive, such as the number of embryos to transfer during IVF or the fate of frozen embryos, will need particularly careful thought.

Support Counselling

The investigation and treatment of infertility are often stressful, as we have seen. So there are times when most people welcome some emotional support, especially after a failed attempt at assisted conception or when treatment is finally to be discontinued. For many couples support will chiefly come from friends and relatives or from a voluntary, perhaps entirely informal, support group. However, many such groups themselves welcome the advice of a counsellor.

Therapeutic Counselling

Therapeutic counselling concentrates on healing, especially in helping the couple adjust to hard circumstances and eventually to accept them. Some people never need counselling; others may need it, if only occasionally, for some years.

5. Infertility Treatments: The First Line

Few couples are wholly infertile, so even after many years of failure some couples will achieve a pregnancy without apparently changing their lifestyle, let alone having treatment. On the other hand, probably fewer than half of the couples who start treatment for their infertility will manage to have a baby as a result. It is therefore vital that couples are told candidly about the limited chances from the outset: it may be equally necessary to help them face the possibility of childlessness as to give the treatment aimed at overcoming it. Many couples have told us that their doctors were so keen to get them pregnant that no one talked about what would happen if they failed – a subject we return to in Chapter 11.

We shall now look at the kinds of treatment available from the family doctor or from District Hospitals, the 'secondary' centres. More complex procedures, like IVF and GIFT, discussed in Chapter 6, are mostly available only from specialized regional units – the 'tertiary' centres – or from private clinics.

Treatment for Men

As we have stressed, over a third of all infertility is wholly or partly due to a problem in the male partner. Yet most kinds of male infertility are difficult to treat and there are no certain ways of increasing sperm counts. The majority of men seem to produce a satisfactory quality and quantity of sperm, regardless of what they do, but provided that there is no fundamental problem such as a chromosome defect or a high level of antibodies, a low sperm count can sometimes be dramatically improved by simple health measures like improving diet and reducing excess weight. Reducing both alcohol intake and smoking can help, as can cutting down on tea and coffee drinking, as caffeine may inhibit the production of sperm.

Regular exercise should improve sperm production, but very strenuous exercise such as marathon running or daily games of squash may be detrimental. A rest from these demanding routines may be all that is needed for a pregnancy to be achieved.

In the case of some high-powered executives, or their over-stretched employees, a change in working patterns may be necessary, but this is easier said than done. Jobs involving the man in a lot of stressful travel may affect sperm production as well as reducing the opportunities for conception, when he is away at crucial times.

Reducing testicular temperature has long been thought to improve sperm production. Wearing looser-fitting underpants, like boxer shorts, instead of Y-fronts is worth a try, although there is no conclusive proof of the efficacy of this. More dramatic methods have been suggested, such as using ice packs during intercourse. This may make love-making more exciting (or divisive!) but is unlikely to affect sperm production.

Drugs

A wide range of drugs has been tried in order to help overcome male infertility, but success rates are said to be very low and in most cases are not only a waste of money but delay the taking of more appropriate action. The only definite indication for drug treatment is a hormone deficiency due to the under-functioning of the pituitary gland. Gonadotrophin replacement may then help sperm production.

Testosterone and synthetic substitutes such as mesterolone

(on the market as Proviron) have been taken by thousands of men, but when pregnancy follows in their female partners there is no proof that it would not have happened anyway and the drug may even decrease sperm production. Steroid drugs, such as prednisolone, have been effective in the small minority of cases where antibodies are found to be damaging the sperm. But steroids produce harmful side-effects and should be given only for short periods and with careful monitoring.

Antibiotic treatment of infection in the testes may greatly improve the sperm count by clearing the inflammation, but couples must remember that the change will not be sudden: it takes about two months for a sperm to mature.

Surgical and Other Treatments

Varicose veins in the testis (varicoceles) can be surgically corrected either by tying off the abnormal vessels or blocking them with an injected chemical. These are safe and simple procedures but there are different views on their effectiveness, though a significant rise in sperm count has been reported in some men.

Unblocking the vas deferens is a more complicated operation as it is done by microsurgery, which requires great skill. Success depends partly on the extent of the blockage. Unfortunately sperm production may have become irreversibly damaged if the blockage has been there for a long time, so many operations, though technically successful, do not assist conception.

Blockages may of course be due to a vasectomy performed when the man did not expect to want another child. In relation to male infertility, reversal of a vasectomy is probably the most common reason for performing surgery, but attempts at reversal after seven years or so are rarely successful.

In some men the problem does not lie in a low or non-existent capacity to produce sperm but in difficulties in achieving an erection and hence coition. This common and distressing problem may be due to physical or psychological causes or both. Various treatments have been developed, including counselling, sexual therapy and such physical aids as pumps. In the great majority of cases the problem can be overcome but help should be sought as early as possible.

Artificial Insemination

Artificial insemination of a woman with her partner's sperm can overcome any problems due to ineffective or absent intercourse. This is known as AIH – artificial insemination by husband. With some techniques this procedure can also bypass disorders of the cervix. For otherwise normal men with low sperm counts, AIH can ensure that a larger number of sperm reach the fallopian tube. Sperm may also be retrieved direct from the testis if the epididymis or vas deferens are blocked, although this has a low success rate as the sperm are immature.

For people having difficulty with intercourse, the semen may be collected after masturbation and deposited untreated near the cervix through a small tube so that the sperm can make their own way into the womb.

If there is an abnormality of the cervix, or, in some cases, a low sperm count, the semen may be injected straight into the womb through a small tube passed through the cervix. Here the semen must be specially prepared in order to avoid risk of infection and to remove prostaglandins – hormones which might otherwise cause contractions of the uterus.

In cases of low sperm count, the semen is treated or 'washed' before insemination to remove any dead or abnormal sperm. Sometimes the man is asked to collect the first part of his ejaculate separately (a method referred to as split ejaculate), as this contains a higher concentration of sperm.

Some men find masturbating under clinical conditions, however private, difficult or stressful and they may be embarrassed by failure to produce a specimen to order. Staff in the clinics are well used to the difficulties and will be very understanding.

If a man knows that he may soon lose his capacity to produce sperm or that the sperm may be damaged by, for instance, anti-cancer drugs or irradiation, the sperm can be collected and frozen for later use by artificial insemination (see Chapter 6).

Donor Insemination (DI)

If none of these treatments enable the man to fertilize his partner, the only way forward may be via artificial insemination using sperm from a donor. This is called DI – donor insemination. Thousands of couples have achieved pregnancies in this way. Despite frequent unease on the couple's part to begin with, an eventually happy result is not uncommon.

Nevertheless it should not be undertaken lightly. The procedure is relatively simple and cheap but the success rate is low and has decreased since it became compulsory to use frozen sperm to avoid the risk of HIV infection. Couples may have to make many attempts.

Ovulation is sometimes stimulated to try to improve the chance of success in DI treatment. So far this has made little difference to the overall chances of having a baby but, not surprisingly, the risk of a multiple pregnancy increases (see Chapter 7).

Couples are bound to dislike the lack of spontaneity and the inevitably clinical approach. Precise timing of ovulation is essential and too many women are told to rely on temperature charts rather than have the necessary monitoring by measuring hormone levels (in urine or blood) or by ultrasound. Thus many attempts are doomed to unnecessary failure and the couples to disappointment. Many give up after only a few months.

Any couple considering using donor sperm will clearly need to think long and hard, probably with the help of a counsellor, about the possible social and psychological implications both for them and any resulting child. How will the husband feel when the baby has characteristics of his wife but not of himself? Is he really ready to relinquish genetic parenthood? He may feel excluded when all attention shifts away from him once DI is chosen. His only role then is to support his partner and, in the effort, he may well suppress his own feelings of grief and failure. Are they as a couple ready to tell other family members, and cope with their possibly hostile and questioning reactions? What if his parents dislike the idea of their grand-child bearing their name but not their genes?

What are the couple's feelings about openness in general and eventually telling the child in particular about the circumstances of his or her conception? If they are not prepared to tell him, how will they cope with carrying the secret? Might one of them angrily burst out with the truth one day?

For some couples in our generally monogamous culture, DI can seem almost like adultery. Yet some recipient couples feel quite differently. As one father said: 'I'd rather have a good chance of having *a* child than no chance of having *my* child.' He went on to have healthy twin daughters.

Some fears can be dealt with at once. In Britain at least, unless some private donation has been arranged, the donor (and genetic father) will be an anonymous man who has been medically assessed and carefully screened for his suitability. He will also have been counselled about the role. Medical students have been a popular and easy source of recruits but there are advantages in the donor already having had children. Not only will he have proved his fertility; he is likely to have more insight into the implications of donation both for himself and for his family.

Essentially the donor must be healthy with a good sperm count and not a known carrier for any genetic disorder. Each donor is screened for sexually transmitted infections, including HIV. In addition samples are now frozen for six months before use in order that the HIV testing can be repeated.

In Britain the HFE Act does not allow the identity of the donor to be revealed to the couple or to any resulting children. It does provide for possible future changes in the regulations, but guarantees that such changes would not be retroactive. Thus a current donor can be confident that his name will never be released.

Even the small amount of information now taken has discouraged some would-be donors out of fear of disclosure or of acquiring some financial responsibility for the child. But provided donor insemination is carried out in a licensed clinic, the donor's anonymity (in Britain) is virtually absolute, as is his exemption from financial responsibility. However, donors who give their sperm in any agreement not sanctioned by a licensed infertility clinic will be regarded legally as the father of the child and as such be liable for financial maintenance.

Many officially recruited donors have proved willing to give extra, self-descriptive (but not identifying) information, for which the children may well be grateful later. Adopted children are often more interested in knowing the characteristics of their genetic parents than their actual identity.

When the law was changed in Sweden to allow the identity of sperm donors to be made known to both mother and child, donations dropped by 75 per cent. For a while many clinics were left sadly short of donors, although numbers are now rising again. The donors, however, are different: many are older and usually already fathers themselves rather than medical students.

Under the British HFE Act of 1990 all potential donors,

male or female, must be counselled about the various implications of donation before giving either gametes or embryos. They need to explore their motives and their feelings about the potential child and about relinquishing knowledge of, let alone responsibility for, their genetic offspring. This is particularly necessary should the donor otherwise remain childless. Donors also need to think about any possible implications for their present or future family. Care is needed since little is known about the effect of donation on donors, partly due to the secrecy inevitably surrounding the subject.

To reduce the danger of any unwitting incest occurring between children fathered by the same donor, many countries limit the number of offspring allowed from a particular donor. In Britain the number is ten, although some think this could be increased provided there is a good geographical spread of the recipients. Occasionally the limit is exceeded (provided the donor has not stipulated an upper limit himself) in order to allow a couple to use the same donor for a subsequent pregnancy. The children can then be genetic siblings rather than half-siblings with only one parent's genes in common.

Donors have sometimes tried to find out about the children they have fathered but, in Britain at least, donors have no statutory right to learn about them and therefore have to prepare themselves for the possibility of remaining insatiably curious. That some men have later regretted their donation reinforces the need for careful counselling and ample time for reflection. Yet most do seem to have been delighted to help infertile couples, and never regret it.

The Child

In the UK registration of DI babies is just the same as for naturally conceived ones unless DI has been given without the male partner's consent. Legally they have the same status as naturally conceived children with the exception of not being allowed to inherit a title. (Since this is not policed, and parents are not bound to tell children of their origins; in any case, this provision is probably ineffectual. Indeed it is an incentive not to tell the child!)

By law children may not be given any identifying details of their donor father but at eighteen may ask the HFEA about his general characteristics. When a donor's child is planning to marry, or to establish an equivalent partnership, he or she may ask the HFEA to check that the partners are not genetically related. Before being given information about the donor, counselling has to be offered to his genetic child about the child's possible reactions to the information, including frustration at being unable to identify or to meet him.

Parents should always be able to contact their treatment centre for advice on issues arising as their children grow up. Children born following DI should themselves have access to a counsellor and may also receive useful advice and support through the (voluntary) DI Network (see Where to Find Help), which was started by parents who believe in telling their children about their origins and who support each other and new couples contemplating donor insemination. A sensitively written book, *My Story*, explains DI in a straightforward way for four- to five-year-olds.[1] Although the concept of DI is inevitably more difficult than adoption for a young child to understand, there is the advantage that no rejection is involved. Indeed the child may be pleased to know how much he or she was wanted.

Both the HFEA and the British Medical Association (BMA) believe parents should be encouraged to be frank with their children about their origins. However, there are many couples who feel the opposite, particularly if DI was resorted to because of the male partner's infertility. What seems crucial is that children should not discover their origins inadvertently from an unguarded remark. Clearly, if the child is not to be told, the parents will need to be extremely careful from the outset about who, if anyone, becomes party to the knowledge.

Some couples appear to think of donation as only a form of treatment and manage to persist in regarding the child as their partner's in every sense. This kind of denial and self-deception is unlikely to be helpful in the long term; nor is the practice of continuing intercourse during DI in order to avoid definite knowledge of paternity.

If DI was given to avoid passing on a genetic disease, such as Huntington's (which causes dementia and is eventually fatal), parents are much more likely to tell the children, not least to reassure them that they and their own children will not be at risk.

Reassuring findings emerged from a small study conducted at the University of Exeter by Robert and Elizabeth Snowden on young adults who had been told about their DI conception. None of them was seriously distressed. Some felt pleased they had been so wanted. None rejected their father; indeed some became closer on realizing the pain he must have suffered.[2]

Children told sensitively about DI later in life will not necessarily be upset by the delay as long as they understand their parents' motives. One woman confided to her mother that she was about to start DI treatment. Only then did the mother reveal that the daughter herself had been conceived following DI. In this case the knowledge came as a reassurance and comfort.

Should we ourselves have had children as a result of donor insemination (or the IVF we actually tried), we believe we would have told them about it as soon as they were able to understand. However, several recent studies from different countries have found that only a minority of parents choose to tell their children, and several psychologists have told us they have changed their minds on the subject. One who embarked on her study of DI families firmly believing in the practice of telling the children, later concluded that the deciding factor should be what the parents are comfortable with and that they should not be pressurized into taking either course of action.

Parents may well need guidance not only on how to tell their children but how to avoid telling them by accident. One researcher described how a mother, in front of her three- and five-year-old, explained to her in detail the reasons why she was not going to tell them. Another mother talked of the procedure of DI in complex scientific terms, assuming that her ten-year-old son would not only fail to understand but would have neither curiosity nor apprehension about the strange content of his mother's conversation. Children can, of course, suspect or even learn much from a mere glance at the wrong moment.

Most of us will have some events in our life which we choose to keep private and hence secret. But now that there is so much exposure in the media of all the latest reproductive technologies, any parent has to be prepared for increasingly penetrating questions from his or her child. Nevertheless some parents do decide upon complete concealment.

Treatment for Women

A woman who has not become pregnant after two years of unprotected and regular intercourse may increase her chances of pregnancy by improving her diet and pattern of life, by smoking less, reducing her intake of alcohol and trying to remove any causes of stress. Better timing of sexual intercourse can help but old recommendations, like abstinence from sex during the infertile period, have been abandoned. Nor is an orgasm essential – nor adopting a particular position during intercourse!

Help with Ovulation

One of the most powerful of the new methods for increasing female fertility is the judicious use of appropriate drugs. (Careless or excessive use can result in a multiple pregnancy with all the distressing problems that this can bring, as we explain in Chapter 8.) The drug most commonly administered is clomiphene citrate (on the market as Clomid or Serophene). This was the first fertility drug to be used – back in the 1960s – and it remains a cheap and effective solution for very many women.

Indeed clomiphene is so easy to prescribe that far too many women are given it inappropriately, sometimes long before they have had sufficient chance to conceive naturally. It is also sometimes prescribed before enough effort has been put into discovering the cause of the difficulty. If the problem lies only with the man or with the patency, or degree of openness, of the woman's fallopian tubes, clomiphene will be useless. It may even be harmful, causing the lining of the womb to thicken and thereby prevent the embryo from implanting. It also acts as an anti-oestrogen, causing a thickening of the mucus of the cervix, which may inhibit the passage of the sperm. Either way, the use of inappropriate treatment will delay reaching the correct diagnosis and hence treatment.

Serious side-effects as a result of using clomiphene are very rare. Taking it can lead to super-ovulation, however, and more than one baby may be conceived. Although studies have demonstrated that clomiphene can induce triplets, many couples are told this is not so. A number of couples attending the MBF's Supertwins Clinic (for parents of triplets or higher multiple births) conceived triplets having received no other treatment than clomiphene. Some of the mothers of triplets (and twins) had not even been told they were receiving a drug that could stimulate ovulation. Several only visited the doctor because they were concerned that their periods were irregular. At least one of them was not wanting to conceive one baby at the time, let alone three!

It is clearly vital that couples are warned of the risk of

multiple births before taking clomiphene or other, stronger, drugs. And careful monitoring should be provided routinely.

Although any side-effects from clomiphene are usually relatively minor, some women do start feeling unwell. If this happens, there are other similar (if more expensive) drugs such as tamoxifen (marketed as Tamofen) and cyclofenil (Rehibin) that can be used.

Human chorionic gonadotrophin (HCG) sometimes used to be administered as an injection mid-cycle to work in conjunction with clomiphene. The timing of this injection is crucial, however, because it can actually inhibit fertilization if given even a few hours too early or too late. Consequently few doctors now prescribe HCG, employing instead one of the more potent hormones.

If ovulation is being prevented due to the presence of high levels of prolactin, tablets of bromocriptine (Parlodel) can be extremely effective in reducing its production, but there is no point in taking them in other circumstances.

Where clomiphene has failed to induce ovulation after a few months of treatment, it may be advisable to go on to the much stronger drug, human menopausal gonadotrophin (HMG – whose trade names are Pergonal or Humegon) or gonadotrophin-releasing hormone (GnRH). The latter is a mixture of the pituitary hormones LH and FSH. The FSH is the active hormone, but as it is expensive to separate it from LH, the two are usually prescribed in combination. In fact pure FSH has not been shown to be any more effective than the two drugs combined, although research into methods of producing a more effective form of pure FSH is continuing.

In the past HMG was given by a series of injections but now treatment using a small battery-operated pump is becoming increasingly popular. The pump releases by injection small amounts of hormone in short regular bursts, mimicking more closely the normal menstrual cycle where the hormone is released in this way from the hypothalamus. The pump is worn inconspicuously by the patient under her clothing, more or less all the time. This technical innovation may reduce the cost of treatment and also allows the woman to proceed uninterrupted with her normal working life.

A similar pump can also be used to administer LH-releasing hormone (LHRH), which is given when the hypothalamus is failing to communicate satisfactorily with the pituitary gland.

Another drug that has recently become popular is a GnRH analogue, buserelin (taken as a nasal spray or by injection), used particularly in IVF procedures but also in combination with HMG treatment. This actually suppresses the function of the ovary but in doing so makes it more receptive to the action of HMG. Recent research shows that the quality of embryos produced after treatment with buserelin is more consistent.

Surgery

Exciting advances have also been made in the surgical treatment of some kinds of female infertility, as in male. Surgery is used in the removal of adhesions around the ovaries or the fallopian tubes and carries a fairly good success rate, depending much on the site of the adhesions and their cause. Surgery may also be necessary to remove fibroids or to correct an abnormal uterus, such as one with a septum down the middle, or a double uterus. The specialist would discuss in detail the operation being recommended in each case.

Blocked fallopian tubes have always been a common cause of infertility but the chances of surgical correction were very small until the recent advent of microsurgery. The success rate has now risen from 10 to nearly 50 per cent in some units. Microsurgery is also now used for removing fibroids from the uterus. It is, however, a real art and needs a great deal of practice. Unfortunately so far there are relatively few enthusiasts for it in the UK, although Professor Robert Winston (who runs a renowned infertility clinic at Hammersmith Hospital) is certainly one.

The most common form of blockage of the tubes occurs at the outer end, near the ovaries, and involves the fimbria. Clearance at this site necessitates a difficult operation, greatly assisted by microsurgery. If the tube is blocked at the end leading into the uterus, the most satisfactory method of treatment is to cut out the damaged portion of the tube and then re-implant the cut end into the womb, again using microsurgery. The success rate can be well over 50 per cent and the risk of an ectopic pregnancy is relatively low.

Recently some surgeons have started operating through a laparoscope. The great advantage is that an incision of the abdomen is thereby avoided so the patient's recovery is quicker. However, laparoscopy can only be used in limited circumstances and by those with special expertise.

One of the main reasons why women seek surgery is for the reversal of a sterilization undertaken at a time when they had not envisaged wanting another child. Now the woman may desperately want a child, possibly with a new partner who has not himself experienced parenthood. A woman may feel guilty if she frustrates his longing. With microsurgery the majority of sterilized women can have their situation reversed, but the success rate of reversal depends on the method originally used for the sterilization. The original surgeon would not, of course, have expected a reversal to be requested.

Egg Donation

If, for whatever reason, a woman cannot produce healthy eggs (or oöcytes) she might well achieve a pregnancy through being given those of another woman. This procedure is not nearly as common or easy as DI but is now well established.

Egg donation is most likely to be considered when the woman is suffering either from ovarian failure, as described in Chapter 4, or is a carrier for a genetic disease such as haemophilia, which she would be in danger of transmitting to her sons. A few women who persistently produce poor-quality oocytes during IVF treatment may also be suitable recipients.

So far three main sources of eggs have been available. One is the eggs found to be surplus to treatment cycles in IVF and GIFT programmes described in the next chapter. (Spare embryos are often produced during IVF too, but these are becoming scarcer as units acquire facilities for freezing and therefore storing embryos for the couple's own use months or years later. The donation of embryos should not be thought of in the same light as the donation of gametes – eggs and sperm. Many couples regard an embryo as their child.)

A second source of eggs has been women who donate them when being sterilized. A third has been women who donate for purely altruistic reasons. Of these a few have been recruited by the would-be recipient, but in such cases the eggs would need to be exchanged with those from another donor so that proper anonymity can be preserved. (The HFEA guidelines concerning the anonymity of egg donors, as of sperm donors, were summarized earlier in this chapter.) A fourth potential source is women who are prepared to sell their eggs. This is not allowed in Britain, partly for fear of eggs being sold by, for example, young women who are addicted to drugs. In the US, however, young women of a specified description at some of the top universities have reportedly been offered up to $5000 and a free week in New York for just one egg (*The Times*, 8 February 1995). Since the infertile couples who place the advertisements insist on a photograph, it is obvious that anonymity is not only impossible but deliberately prevented. Possible, but highly controversial, new sources of eggs or of actual ovarian tissue, such as adult cadavers or aborted fetuses, will be discussed in Chapter 13.

In preparing for the donation of eggs, donors go through similar procedures to those experienced by women undergoing IVF: they receive drugs to stimulate the ovarian follicles, followed by the egg collection as in the first stage of IVF (see Chapter 6). Becoming an egg donor is therefore a substantial commitment and can involve inconvenience in terms of both time and discomfort. As for male donors, preparatory counselling is therefore rightly mandatory in the UK. Because there is inevitably some risk involved for the donor, however small, the counselling has to differ from that for sperm donation and the regulations may need to also.

Hence no one should ever be put under obligation, financial or otherwise, to donate eggs. In the UK and some other countries their sale is illegal. Some private clinics have allegedly offered free abortions to those prepared to donate eggs at the same time or have induced women to give eggs as a part payment for IVF treatment. In such cases, at the very least, the counselling about donation and about the infertility treatment should be clearly separated. We return, in Chapter 13 to some of the moral issues involved in donation.

Incidentally, the success rate of IVF when donated eggs are used is somewhat higher than that of normal IVF – at about 30 per cent per transfer. No doubt this is partly because the eggs often come from younger women.

The ideal donors are women under thirty-five who have completed their families and are being sterilized. Each year 90,000 or so sterilizations are carried out in the UK but few women realize beforehand that they can donate eggs, let alone that the egg collection can be done at the same time. The National Egg and Embryo Donation Society (NEEDS) seeks to raise public awareness of the unsatisfied demand for eggs and of the potential for egg donation. They also put would-be donors in touch with their nearest donor centre.

Alternative Therapies

We know of no formal studies on the effectiveness of treating infertility using alternative therapies, such as homeopathy, acupuncture, hypnotherapy and herbalism, but we have no doubt that they have a place. A number of the practitioners have told us of couples they have treated successfully after years of failure using conventional remedies. Many of these alternative therapies focus on the overall physical and mental health of the patients by improving their diet, correcting their metabolic balance (and any deficiences such as zinc) and encouraging relaxation.

Many couples feel their general health and equanimity has improved, as in our own case, without the treatment necessarily leading to the conception of a baby.

6. The New Reproductive Technologies

Many infertile couples only have a serious chance of producing a child if they can obtain one of the new forms of assisted conception like IVF or GIFT. This is certainly true if donated eggs have to be used. (Artificial insemination can in practice be do-it-yourself, though we are far from recommending this.)

Before describing the new techniques and their many variations, we should outline the way in which patients are selected and their chances of obtaining these more involved and expensive kinds of treatment. Selection is much less problematic than provision which, in the UK – unlike most West European countries – is sorely inadequate for those unable to pay.

Selection

Other things being equal, infertility specialists will generally be prepared to give the appropriate treatment to any healthy (and non-addicted), settled couple, married or not, who have a reasonable chance of a successful pregnancy and are likely to prove adequate parents. There will be approximate age limits for receiving some forms of treatment, and those that have already had a child, albeit by a different partner, will not be given as high a priority as those who have not.

Doctors naturally differ somewhat in the way they apply these criteria, as they will in their attitude towards, for example, applicants who are single or lesbians (to be discussed in Chapter 14). Quite plainly no competent doctor should knowingly recommend or administer a form of treatment inappropriate to the medical condition of the couple in question. Nevertheless IVF treatment is sometimes given without sufficient prior investigation to see if such a complex and expensive procedure is really necessary, or indeed whether a pregnancy would be likely to be sustained. Choosing between some forms of treatment may not always be easy, especially when the infertility is unexplained, but any areas of medical doubt should be discussed frankly with the couple concerned in the light of their medical history and after proper diagnostic tests.

Availability of Treatment

Doctors do not operate in a purely medical vacuum. Availability of treatment, and therefore money, will enter the equation. Where couples are able and willing to pay, there are many private clinics willing to provide whatever kind of treatment is thought appropriate, subject only to the requirements of medical ethics and any law, such as the British HFE Act of 1990.

Access to treatment, including private treatment, varies hugely between countries, even provinces, as does its affordability. Estimating the costs of infertility treatment can be quite complex, even contentious. Many will see the cost per successful delivery as more relevant than the cost of an individual treatment cycle. A study in the US based on figures for 1992 (when the cost of a single IVF cycle was taken as $8,000) estimated that the average cost per live delivery was $66,667 for the first cycle of IVF. But this cost had risen to $114,286 by the sixth cycle. For women with a good chance of success, such as those with tubal disease, the figures were $50,000 for the first cycle and $72,727 for the sixth. In women who were older, where there was also male infertility to be taken into account, the cost rose from $160,000 for the first cycle to $800,000 for the sixth.[1]

These costs are very high indeed, but they would be far

smaller in the UK and other Western European countries. We have quoted them only to demonstrate the relative costs of a series of IVF treatments compared with that of a single course of IVF leading to a live birth.

In the less-developed world immense numbers of people will scarcely have heard of many of the types of treatment and could not obtain them if they had. Infertility is a global phenomenon and is at least as prevalent and painful in poor societies as in rich ones. (The causes of infertility appear to be broadly the same worldwide, although tubal damage is more common in Africa owing to a high incidence of sexually transmitted pelvic infection.)

Choosing a Clinic

For couples able and willing to take the private route to treatment, the family doctor or hospital gynaecologist will be able to suggest a suitable clinic or wholly specialized infertility centre. The HFEA also issues leaflets and lists of addresses, as do ISSUE and CHILD (see Where to Find Help).

Many people think that figures relating to the outcome of each kind of treatment in each individual centre, private or public, should be made generally available to help would-be clients make their own informed judgement as to the type and place of treatment. At present such figures are confidential to the HFEA, and few clinics publish their own. (There are admittedly many difficulties both in defining 'success rates' and in making comparisons between particular clinics that may take on couples of varying ages and sorts of problem.) Every centre should be ready to answer direct questions from prospective clients or their doctor, and all such information should be made easily available for scrutiny and comparison. However, the interpretation of such figures, and their relevance to any given individual case, remains hard to assess.

Public Provision in the UK

The greatest difficulties arise for couples unable to pay for their own treatment and therefore dependent on a national health service. In many European countries the state will pay most or all of the cost. In Britain the situation is much less satisfactory.

Many District Health Authorities appear to regard infertility as of low priority, failing to recognize that couples may be profoundly distressed or depressed by a condition at once medically caused and genuinely disabling. Few Authorities offer the more expensive forms of treatment that many couples need. Some Authorities, Hospital Trusts and NHS clinics are trying to be as enlightened and effective as wider circumstances allow, but overall the system is eccentrically variable, as between different areas, and grossly inadequate.

Most District Hospitals do not have a specialized infertility clinic and have to depend on their general gynaecology clinic. Perhaps inevitably, these tend to lack sufficient expertise, time and resources to offer complex, expensive or new methods of infertility diagnosis and management. Unless one of the consultants is especially motivated and well provided for, the patient's best hope will be to get access to one of the tertiary regional centres which have specialized clinics offering vital counselling services as well as research and teaching.

Some tests are straightforward, inexpensive and readily provided by the family doctor or District Hospital. This also applies to some forms of treatment. But if the problem is at all obscure, there may well be long delays before the couple see an appropriate consultant and then obtain the relevant tests, possibly a succession of them, followed by a diagnosis. If ovulation proves to be the problem, treatment with clomiphene, or its equivalent, should be readily forthcoming. If, however, some form of assisted conception is needed, most British couples will currently have to turn to the private sector.

NHS centres, whether District Hospitals or tertiary centres, will be much more selective than private clinics about which couples they take on. The chance of getting any particular kind of treatment may depend on the special interests of the consultants or their research programmes, which may be microsurgery, operative laparoscopy, hysteroscopy or one of the new drug therapies. This specialization is understandable when money is tight and staff limited, but so is the annoyance of a couple whose problem is considered less interesting.

NHS medical staff are naturally keen to extend as well as develop their work. Nor should anyone envy health managers their need to decide medical priorities. In relation to assisted conception, various approaches have been employed in order to square the circle. Since payment for NHS treatment as such is barred, its provision is often now funded by charging patients who are accorded 'private patient' status. Under this sort of scheme the patient is charged as a user of an NHS hospital 'private patient facility' to cover the costs of space, equipment, infrastructure, staff and consumables, but not for the consultant's services. This is said to have worked well for some years at the John Radcliffe Hospital, Oxford – a tertiary centre – at a cost to patients of about half of what is commonly charged by private clinics.

Assisted Conception

Treatment by assisted conception replaces the normal method of fertilization rather than just enhancing the couple's capacity to produce sufficient healthy eggs or sperm. In this sense it is not a way of treating infertility so much as a procedure for getting round it. The patient remains 'infertile' but does have the joy of producing a child or children.

Since the birth of Louise Brown in 1978, many thousands more 'test-tube' babies have been born in the UK and most other developed countries. Ever more sophisticated methods of assisted conception have continued to be developed, some of which we now outline.

Assisted conception may be attempted for a number of reasons: to bypass blocked or damaged fallopian tubes; to employ concentrated sperm where their quantity or quality is poor; to assist the sperm to penetrate the egg; or to enable the use of donor gametes where the couple's egg or sperm are unsuitable. It has also been used successfully in many cases of unexplained infertility.

Current Procedures

IVF (*In Vitro Fertilization*) or IVF-ET (*In Vitro Fertilization and Embryo Transfer*)

As previously stated, this is sometimes known as the 'test-tube' method, although no test-tube as such is used. In essence the egg is fertilized in a dish and the resulting embryo transferred into the uterus, usually after two days.

IVF was originally devised for women whose fallopian tubes were damaged or blocked, but is now increasingly used for couples with other conditions such as endometriosis, low sperm counts, immunological problems such as antibodies that damage sperm, and for couples where their infertility is unexplained.

By showing whether the egg is fertilized in the dish, this technique also serves as a test of the partner's sperm. Some clinics are therefore now employing a complete first IVF treatment as at once a test and a first attempt at an induced pregnancy. If the 'test' also produces a pregnancy, few patients will complain. This approach should also reduce the overall cost of diagnosis and treatment, but it will not be appropriate in all cases.

In 1992, 13,791 women received a total of 18,224 treatment cycles in the UK, of which the overwhelming majority took place in private clinics rather than through the NHS.

Before embarking on IVF the specialist will always explain the procedure and ensure that the couple receive appropriate advice and counselling, as described in Chapter 4.

The four-week treatment cycle involves four main stages. First the ovaries are stimulated with drugs so that more than the usual single egg will mature and become available for retrieval. This usually involves the woman having hormone injections, blood tests to measure the hormone levels during the first half of the cycle, and ultrasound scans to monitor the growth of the follicles in the ovary. From the results of these tests the specialist determines the best time to perform the egg collection, which is after the eggs have matured but before they are released from the ovaries.

Second comes the egg collection, which may be done under sedation or a general anaesthetic, using ultrasound monitoring through the vagina or the abdomen. A hollow needle is introduced into the abdomen and an egg sucked out (aspirated) from each accessible mature follicle in the ovary. Some specialists prefer to aspirate the eggs under direct vision, so do this via a laparoscope inserted through a small incision below the navel or umbilicus.

The eggs are next incubated in a culture medium for a few hours. The partner then produces (in private) some semen by masturbation, and when the motile sperm have been concentrated, this prepared semen is added to the culture medium with the eggs. Fertilization takes about eighteen hours and it is another twelve hours before the cells start to divide. After forty-eight hours, when they have each divided into two to four cells, they are ready for transfer to the woman's uterus.

Finally, if more than three eggs have been fertilized, no more than three of the most healthy ones are loaded into a very fine catheter. This is passed through the cervix and the embryos deposited at the top of the uterus. (Some countries permit the transfer of more than three embryos, but this is the legal limit in the UK. Indeed some units transfer only two embryos to younger women, for fear of creating triplets.)

The couple then go home to wait, and hope. There is no evidence that they can do anything special to enhance the chances of an embryo becoming implanted. Most specialists recommend that the woman resumes her normal activities.

In a few cases treatment will have to be abandoned at some stage during the cycle. This may be due to poor response to the ovulation-stimulating drugs, to difficulty in retrieving the eggs or because no egg has been fertilized. With improved methods the percentage of abandoned cycles is now much smaller than it used to be.

GIFT (Gamete Intra-fallopian Transfer)

Conception can be facilitated by adding the man's sperm to a fluid containing his partner's eggs and transferring them together and directly to the fallopian tubes at the most favourable time in the menstrual cycle. Thus although the conception is still assisted, it does occur inside the woman. GIFT is practised in most units which undertake IVF and in a number that do not.

GIFT can only be employed when the patient has at least one fallopian tube that is open, or patent. Specialists vary greatly in their enthusiasm for the procedure, but many employ it in cases of unexplained infertility.

The initial stages of the GIFT treatment cycle are the same as for IVF, until the point at which the eggs have been recovered. Once all the eggs have been collected, a preparation of the partner's sperm is drawn into a fine tube, together with up to three eggs. The tube is usually introduced through a laparoscope into the abdomen and gently inserted into the outer end of one or both fallopian tubes, into which the sperm and eggs are flushed. This method is also sometimes employed for DI.

ZIFT (*Zygote Intra-fallopian Transfer*) or PROST (*Pronuclear Oocyte Stage Transfer*)

This procedure is the same as IVF except that the fertilized egg is transferred a few hours earlier and into the fallopian tube rather than into the uterus, thereby mimicking a natural pregnancy more closely. The eggs are introduced through a laparoscope into the open end of the fallopian tube, which must of course be patent. In practice ZIFT is mainly used where there is male infertility. The advantage over GIFT is that fertilization can be seen to have taken place before the transfer is effected.

TEST (*Tubal Embryo Stage Transfer*) or TET (*Tubal Embryo Transfer*)

This procedure is the same as ZIFT except that the transfer is delayed until the fertilized eggs have divided into two or more cells.

POST (*Peritoneal Oocyte and Sperm Transfer*)

The first two stages of POST are the same as for IVF. Up to three eggs are then mixed with a prepared sample of 'washed' sperm and injected into the cavity of the abdomen just behind the uterus, known as the Pouch of Douglas. POST has been used in cases of unexplained infertility but also where donor insemination has failed or where patients produce antibodies that damage the sperm. The laboratory work involved with IVF and embryo transfer is not necessary and no anaesthetic is required.

DOT (*Direct Oocyte Transfer*)

This relatively new procedure is similar to IVF except that the eggs are transferred as soon as a sperm is seen to be attached to the egg, but before fertilization has taken place.

TUFT (*Trans-uterine Fallopian Transfer*)

This procedure is similar to ZIFT but has the advantage that no laparoscopy is needed as the embryo is transferred to the fallopian tube through a soft plastic canula which is introduced through the cervix into the uterus and then threaded up the fallopian tube. This is a recently developed technique and it is too early to judge its usefulness.

MAF (*Micro-assisted Fertilization*)

IVF sometimes fails because the sperm fails to penetrate the outer shell of the egg, the zona pellucida. To assist penetration a number of MAF techniques have been devised:

1. PZD (partial zona dissection): Here the outer shell can be punctured (known as zona puncture) or torn (zona tearing) so that a sperm is more likely to find its way through to fertilize the egg. Once fertilization has occurred, the procedure is the same as for IVF.

2. SUZI (sub-zonal insemination): Where the sperm still fails to penetrate, single sperm can now be picked up by a glass micro-needle and deposited just beneath the shell of the egg. A new technique known as CISS (computer-image sperm selection) has been devised for selecting the best sperm. The Hobson sperm tracker, based on the latest motor traffic 'eye', is used to compute the special movement co-ordinates of the stronger sperm and these are tracked on a monitor before being picked out using a needle said to be seven times thinner than a human hair.

3. ICSI (intra-cytoplasmic sperm injection) or DISCO (direct injection of sperm into the cytoplasm of the oocyte): In ICSI (or DISCO) a single sperm is deposited in the cytoplasm surrounding the nucleus of the egg so that it bypasses all the normal barriers that sperm have to encounter. It could therefore be used when none of the sperm have normal motility and where only a very few sperm are available.

Some experts regard ICSI as an historic breakthrough in

treating male infertility. Others are uneasy about a procedure that circumvents all natural selective barriers to fertilization, including the competition of stronger sperm. They fear that defective genes may be introduced inadvertently which will be passed on to the child. They also fear that the injection process might itself harm the sperm or egg, or introduce foreign substances such as bits of the egg's outer coating or even infection. So far (from admittedly few cases) there has been no evidence of this happening, but the treatment should clearly be confined to centres with facilities for full monitoring and follow-up of the resulting children as well as the appropriate technical expertise.

ICSI is a new medical technique in respect of humans, although it has been used by animal embryologists since the 1960s. It is normally only employed after SUZI has failed as it is the most invasive procedure of all. In 1994 the HFEA granted the first licence for ICSI to be performed as a clinical service.

MESA (Microsurgical Epididymal Sperm Aspiration)
When there is a blockage to the male duct system, sperm can be collected from the epididymis and then introduced by artificial insemination.

IUI (Intra-uterine Insemination)
Sperm that need special preparation can be placed within the cavity of the uterus by intra-uterine insemination (IUI). This is used in cases of low sperm counts and often in conjunction with hyperstimulation of the ovaries.

DIPI (Direct Intra-peritoneal Insemination)
This has been used for couples with unexplained infertility, sperm-damaging antibodies, low sperm counts and for whom donor insemination has failed. The first steps are similar to those taken in the preliminary stage of an IVF cycle. When the

follicles are judged to be mature, a washed sample of semen is injected through the top of the vagina into the cavity of the abdomen in the Pouch of Douglas. The sperm are then wafted into the fallopian tube, together with the eggs as they are released from the ovaries. The success rate is relatively low, so DIPI is usually undertaken only where more sophisticated methods are not available.

The Donation of Gametes

All the various forms of assisted conception so far described in this chapter can be employed with either the couple's own gametes (sperm or eggs) or with donated gametes (see Chapter 5).

Cryopreservation

Embryos can be stored for long periods at very low temperatures and this cryopreservation can be a method of assisting conception in some cases. In 1992 frozen embryos were used in 2,307 IVF treatment cycles (about 13 per cent of the total number). Many units now provide cryopreservation facilities where surplus embryos can be frozen for use in the future. (Legal controls vary from country to country – see Chapter 15.)

The main reasons for freezing are first to preserve eggs or sperm which might otherwise be irreversibly damaged by medical treatment such as chemotherapy or radiation, or where the ovaries or testes are to be removed because of disease. Secondly freezing enables embryos that are surplus in a particular IVF treatment cycle to be preserved, thereby permitting the woman to make later IVF attempts within a normal menstrual cycle without requiring more ovarian stimulation. And, finally, cryopreservation allows time for the donors of gametes to be screened for infection and, in the case of HIV, to have a second test before the sperm or eggs are used.

Cryopreservation of eggs is less satisfactory than that of embryos as the egg is particularly sensitive to temperature. This is unfortunate as many people feel more comfortable about the freezing of gametes than of embryos.

Enthusiasm for the use of frozen embryos varies greatly, as does the success rate. Some specialists feel their use should be restricted to women for whom no fresh eggs are available, at least until more is known about the long-term health and development of the resulting children. There has been no evidence of problems so far but the first children to be produced are all still very young.

Disturbing questions can arise for the couple if they successfully complete their family without needing all their stored embryos. The embryos could then be discarded, given to another couple, used for research or continue to be stored (in the UK for up to five years and usually at considerable cost to the couple) but without expectation that they will ever be used.

Some couples we have met have said they were distressed and bewildered when faced with deciding between these options. 'The agonizing choice: do we let our "babies" die?' was one headline. One mother who attends the MBF's Twins Clinic was horrified to find that her surplus eggs from a GIFT treatment cycle had been fertilized (by her partner's sperm), without her permission, before being frozen and stored. She felt the decision as to their final disposal, five years later, was made much harder because she saw these embryos as her children, which potentially of course they were.

Surrogacy

It can be peculiarly painful for would-be parents to produce good eggs and sperm yet prove unable to nurture an embryo because the womb is absent or damaged. Throughout history couples have overcome childlessness by finding a woman, sometimes a sister, who is willing to bear a child for them. Since the advent of IVF and GIFT, full surrogacy or 'host mothering' has become possible, whereby the host mother gestates an embryo that is the genetic offspring of both partners. An alternative course employs the surrogate's own eggs and is known as 'straight surrogacy'. The surrogate's egg or eggs may be fertilized following natural or artificial insemination with the male partner's sperm or indeed a donor's.

Under British law surrogacy is permissible but advertising is illegal (whether for or by surrogates) and surrogate mothers are not allowed to be paid for their service, as opposed to being refunded their full expenses. These expenses are commonly assessed as being £10,000 or more. The main reason for banning the sale as such of surrogacy has been to discourage unsuitable or unhealthy women from offering their services, including drug addicts desperate to get money for drugs.

Nevertheless some experts feel that proper remuneration (combined with rigorous health checks) would be more appropriate because the surrogate's motives would be more straightforward and emotionally disinterested, and hence more stable. As it is legitimate for clinics to provide assisted conception for profit, it is not entirely clear why they or some other bodies should not facilitate surrogacy on a commercial basis, provided always that proper health checks and other necessary preconditions, including counselling, are fulfilled.

One non-medical organization offers information, advice and support. This is COTS (Childlessness Overcome Through Surrogacy), a voluntary organization founded by Kim Cotton, the surrogate mother whose story caused tabloid mania about ten years ago.

Surrogacy is currently not regulated in the UK and many feel that it should be brought under the jurisdiction of the HFEA and that any agencies facilitating it should be licensed.

At present an agency can be run by a surrogate mother herself. Nor are there any controls on the suitability of would-be surrogates.

Many surrogates have received no counselling and been ill-prepared for the bereavement they have felt on handing over the baby. One surrogate mother was shattered to find that she was carrying a baby with Down's syndrome and that the parents wanted her to have a termination of the pregnancy despite her own deep reluctance. The number of surrogacies that have failed in one way or another does not appear to be high, although there is as yet no reliable knowledge of its frequency.

Most surrogacy is carried out by friends and relatives. In the UK about 120 cases of surrogacy are recorded each year, but many more are known to occur without being formally reported. The true figure is more likely to be about 300.

In 1994 triplets were successfully brought to birth by a woman after IVF treatment using embryos produced by her brother and sister-in-law. This caused quite a stir, but back in 1987 a South African Catholic woman had already given birth to surrogate triplets, and at the age of forty-eight. Moreover these triplets were in fact her own genetic grandchildren, in that the embryo derived from her own daughter who had been left barren at the age of twenty-two, following the birth of her only son.

Such cases cause many people serious unease, but they tend to be more worried where the transaction is not between members of the same family and where the motive is therefore less personal and there may be risks of damage from separating the child and the gestatory mother. In some cases, however, the surrogate mother becomes a friend and we know of at least one who has twice borne children for the same couple – a singleton and then twins.

That serious problems could arise is clear. So, therefore, is the need for careful selection of those involved and supervision of the arrangements entailed. Nevertheless, in general, medical and public opinion seems to be becoming more sympathetic to surrogacy, not least because the tragedy of premature hysterectomies, and the like, is now more widely appreciated. There have even been cases of successful surrogate pregnancies being achieved for would-be parents following the use of genetically unrelated embryos left over from another couple's treatment. This also opens up the possibility of using the would-be father's sperm and a donated egg, or using donated embryos stored in a 'bank'. The ethical controversies seem unlikely to subside.

7. The Outcomes of Treatment

The Chances of Success

It would be enormously helpful to infertile couples if they could be given a reliable estimate of their chances of achieving a successful pregnancy. Yet crude pregnancy rates per couple would be almost meaningless: we need estimates of the chances of pregnancy for particular diagnoses and sorts of treatment. Even more importantly, we need to know the proportion that lead first to pregnancy and then to the birth of a healthy baby.

The rates for pregnancy or live births should also relate to a defined number of cycles, preferably three or four (after which the success rate tends to fall). Any given couple will hope for at least a rough guide. They have probably been trying for some years and the woman may already be in her late thirties. Chances of only 10 or 20 per cent over a period of two years may seem disappointingly slim, but that could well be the relevant time frame for the couple's decision making.

Some of the difficulties in assessing the chances are worth looking at more closely. All couples are different. Sometimes both partners will have physical problems. Some may also have psycho-sexual or other difficulties undetected by the gatherer of statistics. In many couples, as we know ourselves, the infertility remains altogether unexplained. It may remain wholly hidden: many couples never seek help or prefer to remain childless. Some, on the other hand, may become pregnant naturally, if late, while undergoing treatment. No doubt some succeed despite the treatment.

The practical obstacles to properly controlled random studies are clearly manifold and some methods would be ethically unacceptable. In any particular area of treatment a dependable (and comparable) assessment of the results of the treatment will hinge not only on reliable judgement but standardized criteria as to admission, diagnosis, methods and outcomes. Despite all the difficulties, however, several studies have been made and some rough indications of the chances of pregnancy can be attempted. An overview of the situation in the UK may be useful first.

In Britain at least 10 per cent of couples have difficulty in achieving a pregnancy or in going on to have a liveborn child. The proportion of couples experiencing difficulty at some stage or other is generally thought to be as high as one in six. National conception rates and birth rates have risen and fallen in recent years. Much of the variation has been due to people's changing wishes, but access to family planning and abortion have also been influential.

Many pregnancies, indeed a large minority, do not result in a registrable live or still birth. Between 1985 and 1987 only 76 per cent of registered British pregnancies did so. Terminations defined as legal under the 1967 Abortion Act amounted to 17 per cent, and ectopic pregnancies and spontaneous miscarriages made up the remaining 7 per cent of failures.

Yet these figures do not include early miscarriages or cases where there is no hospital admission. It seems likely that a large proportion of pregnancies are lost without the woman even realizing that she was pregnant. Charles Boklage, a scientist in North Carolina, has estimated that only a quarter of pregnancies end up with a live baby, the great majority being lost within the first few weeks after conception. Twin pregnancies are even more vulnerable: only 2 per cent end up with two babies and another 12 per cent produce only a single survivor.[1]

The cumulative 'take-home' baby rates are, of course, what matter most because they give some indication of what might prove possible after a number of cycles of treatment. Based on results from several developed countries, Professor Michael Hull of Bristol University suggests a rate of some 60 per cent after four cycles of IVF treatment and higher figures for combinations of methods of assisted conception where there have been six or more cycles. After nine cycles up to 90 per cent have been successful – a very remarkable statistic, if an expensive one.

But such high figures should be treated with great caution. For example, all the women in the Bristol study were under forty, their partners had normal sperm counts and some, as mentioned, had been through many (expensive) IVF cycles. Interpretation also depends on the types of infertility present in these women. Ideally results will gradually be classified by diagnostic category, age and so on.

However, figures on outcomes are difficult to come by because of the imprecise definition of infertility and the wide assortment of cases and forms of treatment. In the UK, for example, no figures have been collected on the prevalence and outcomes of the most common treatment, the use of ovulation-stimulating drugs. Thus we cannot estimate the proportion of couples using them who then succeed. Furthermore, as we have already remarked, many couples are given this and other types of treatment unnecessarily and would have become pregnant anyway.

For treatments that are licensed (such as IVF and DI), the outcomes have to be recorded by law. Even so, the results vary greatly according to the client's age, type of problem and general state of health. They also vary according to the size of the clinic. Large centres (giving more than 400 IVF treatment cycles per year) tend to have higher success rates than medium-sized ones (100–400 treatment cycles), although these in turn do better than small ones. A number of small clinics do nevertheless have high success rates.

The Outcomes of IVF

It is an inevitably slow process compiling national figures, but in the UK, in 1992, just over 18,224 IVF treatment cycles were recorded. Both the pregnancy rate and the live-birth rate have steadily increased since figures first became available in 1985. The pregnancy rate per IVF treatment cycle rose from 11.2 per cent in 1985 to 16.9 per cent in 1992, and the live-birth rate rose from 8.6 to 12.7 per cent in the same period. (The difference between pregnancy rate and live-birth rate is largely due to miscarriage in the first three months of the pregnancy.)

The number of embryos transferred influences the overall success rate and also the multiple-pregnancy rate. In 1991, 60.4 per cent of the transfers were of three embryos and produced a total pregnancy rate of 27 per cent. In that same year 26.3 per cent of the transfers were of two embryos and resulted in a total pregnancy rate of 22.3 per cent. The remaining 13.3 per cent of the transfers were of one embryo and the pregnancy rate for these was only 8.6 per cent. However, some units have had equally good pregnancy rates when transferring two embryos compared to three.

The multiple-pregnancy rate following IVF or GIFT has remained remarkably high even after the UK maximum of three embryos was imposed. Indeed the rate is so high that we have devoted a whole section (Chapter 8) to multiple pregnancy. Anyone embarking on either procedure should first give this possibility serious consideration.

With IVF, as with other forms of treatment, a woman's age greatly affects her chances of a successful outcome. In 1991 the live-birth rate per transfer was 22.1 per cent in the 25–29 age group, compared with 15.2 per cent in the 35–39 age group. For those between forty and forty-four years of age the rate was 8.2 per cent and for those of forty-five and over it was 3.4 per cent.

The picture changes dramatically when donor eggs are used for older women. In the 40–44 age group the chances of a live birth for each treatment cycle was 4.5 per cent using their own eggs but 12.7 per cent with eggs donated by younger women. In the forty-five and over group the respective figures were 1.7 and 17.7 – an immense difference.

The Outcomes of GIFT

In 1991 about 2,000 GIFT treatment cycles were recorded in the UK and the overall success rates were similar to those for IVF with a pregnancy rate per treatment cycle of 17.2 per cent and a live-birth rate of 11.3 per cent. Of the live births, 76.1 per cent were singletons, 18.9 per cent twins, 4.4 per cent triplets and 0.6 per cent quads.

The Outcomes of Donor Insemination

National figures relating to the outcomes of donor insemination have been collected in the UK only since 1991. In 1992 over 4,000 couples received DI, with a clinical pregnancy rate of 6.7 per cent per treatment cycle and a live-birth rate of 5 per cent. The multiple-pregnancy rate varied according to whether ovulation had been stimulated during the cycle. For stimulated cycles the multiple-pregnancy rate was 13.5 per cent and the multiple-birth rate 15.3 per cent. For unstimulated cycles the rates were 1.7 and 2 respectively. (The multiple-birth rate was higher than the multiple-pregnancy rate because a larger proportion of single pregnancies ended in a miscarriage than did multiple pregnancies.) There were ten sets of triplets and one of quads in the stimulated cycles.

In the past, when fresh sperm were used, pregnancy rates following DI were higher and similar to those of the general population. However, since it became compulsory to use sperm that has been frozen (in order to screen for HIV infection), pregnancy rates have fallen.

Weighing up the Chances

To any particular couple the specialist can only offer an informed guess about their own chances of a pregnancy. In addition the same estimate will mean different things to different couples, depending on their own disposition, situation or previous expectations. Optimists will see no reason why they should not be one of the minority who succeed; the pessimist will focus on the majority who fail.

Sooner or later many couples will have to ask themselves the painful question 'How long do we go on trying?' In 1991 seventy-four people then undergoing IVF treatment had been through ten or more treatment cycles; and even then a few couples will produce a baby. We know of one couple who did so after trying seventeen times. Another, in Belgium, had triplets after twenty-three IVF attempts, and an Israeli woman was reported in the *Jewish Chronicle* (9 December 1994) as 'twenty-fifth time lucky' when, at the age of forty-six, she produced boy triplets.

For each of the first four attempts, the chances of a baby remain remarkably similar, ranging from 17.8 to 20.4 per cent. Only on the fifth and later attempts is there a steady decline in the success rate. (A similar pattern is seen with DI – a distinctly higher success rate among the first five attempts than subsequently.)

The very hope that is implicit in the new technologies can drive one to making further attempts. Couples may continue striving for much longer than they would have done in the past, perhaps fearing that failure to pursue every possibility, however remote or expensive, would suggest lack of commitment. Many become exhausted by the struggle. As one woman put it: 'I'm so tired of this. I wish I didn't even want children.'

For those who do not produce a child, merely having tried can give a feeling of accomplishment. One woman who produced three embryos at her first IVF attempt, but remained childless and finally gave up after eight years, described how thrilled she was 'just to know that I was capable of producing potential babies, the thrill of seeing them on the screen. Feelings of hope and overwhelming emotion.'

Couples come to a point when they must weigh the slim remaining chances of success against the emotional, financial and other costs of persisting, not least the strains on their own relationship. Childlessness is not a fate worse than death, as we show in Chapter 11.

Pregnancy

For previously infertile couples pregnancy means a first basic success, and most assume that this will bring them unadulterated elation. For some it certainly does, as for a woman who attempted IVF after seven years of infertility: 'I made my husband take the call, and the delight and supreme joy in his shout told me everything I needed to know. We couldn't believe it, we really couldn't. I went around hugging my tummy for days. When a little later a scan revealed it was twins, we thought we had died and gone to heaven.'

Other couples may feel ambivalent. Pregnancy may be both a blessing and the cause of new concerns. As the years of infertility go by, many women increasingly concentrate on becoming pregnant and may almost forget the original aim of having a child. One mother, who became pregnant after her first IVF attempt, described this vividly.

One's whole being is focused upon becoming pregnant. People who have experienced little difficulty would say: how ridiculous; of course you must become pregnant before you can have a family. But they have no idea how obsessed one can become with the getting pregnant bit. Obsessed to the point of not seeing further – or daring to see further; hence my state of near panic when I had reached the point of having to see further.

It is not unusual for couples to have feelings of panic when the responsibility of caring for a baby becomes a real possibility, indeed probability. The pregnancy can also reactivate doubts and anxieties which have been put aside in the effort to become pregnant. Will all the effort prove worthwhile? The years of trying can build up quite unrealistic expectations of the joys of motherhood.

Some women who have conceived out of the blue after they had stopped trying have actually felt cheated. They feel the pregnancy has arrived too late: they have worked through their grief and bereavement, accepted their loss and even convinced themselves that they no longer wanted motherhood. For some, not having a straightforward single pregnancy can be disappointing. A mother of healthy eight-month-old twin girls described her feelings in the *Prospect Newsletter* of October 1992.

I had never dreamed that we would have twins. I knew with two embryos replaced it could easily happen, but not to me! It was a big shock; my mother said, 'Oh dear.' . . . I found myself thinking that all I ever wanted was to be a normal family with one baby at a time . . . Throughout our eight years of infertility, I had dreamed of how it would be when I became pregnant. How happy I would be and how I would glow. I felt horrible! I suffered nausea, sinusitis, light-headedness, off my food, popping ears, heartburn, breathlessness. In fact every symptom in the book . . . I had hoped to deliver naturally but had to have a Caesarean section . . . I was terribly disappointed as I did not want to miss out on anything, particularly if this was to be my only pregnancy.

Many women feel very anxious during the first stage of their precious pregnancy. They have had plenty of time to learn about the complications that can arise, especially in older women. The risk of having a baby with Down's syndrome or some other abnormality also increases with age. Nevertheless the chances remain low. A 35 to 40-year-old mother has only a one-in-300 chance of having a baby with Down's syndrome.

On the positive side, women who have had difficulty in conceiving are often more accepting of the discomforts and inconveniences of pregnancy. They may be much more tolerant of the frustrations and irritations of visiting antenatal clinics. Familiarity with medical procedures also makes the physical examinations and high technology involved seem less threatening.

One advantage of artificial conception is that there is little doubt about when it took place and therefore about the likely duration of the pregnancy. A pregnancy can be confirmed within two weeks of fertilization, although at this early stage, like any pregnancy, it is still very vulnerable to miscarriage. In pregnancies following IVF about 17 per cent result in miscarriage – a considerably higher rate than normal. This is largely due to the higher average age of the women being treated and to more of them having something physically wrong with them.

In a further 2–3 per cent of cases the pregnancy will be ectopic. This is the potentially dangerous situation in which the embryo implants itself outside the womb (usually in one of the fallopian tubes). It occurs about five times more often in assisted than in normal conceptions because the fallopian tubes are more likely to be damaged and therefore to impede the embryo's passage to the womb.

The danger to the woman arises because the tube may rupture as the fetus grows. She may feel pain and there is often bleeding. This can lead to a surgical emergency where there is no alternative but to end the pregnancy by removing the fetus or by injecting it so that it dies (and shrinks). Very occasionally a twin pregnancy may result in one embryo being implanted in a fallopian tube and the other in the womb: as long as the ectopic embryo is removed, the other baby can develop normally.

Several studies have shown that Caesarean sections are more common in mothers who have had IVF, even when multiple births are taken into account. We have talked to a number of obstetricians who feel this is partly due to the increased anxiety of both the parents and their doctors.

Are there objective grounds for this anxiety? In general it seems that children born following treatment for infertility are as healthy as any others. It is true that the perinatal mortality – that is, babies who are stillborn or who die in the first week of life – among babies produced by assisted conception is about twice that in the general population. This may sound alarming so needs putting into perspective. The most likely explanation is the higher proportion of multiple pregnancies and hence higher degree of prematurity and low birthweight (see Chapter 8). In any case, the actual chances of stillbirth or early death, in absolute terms, remain low.

The first large study of 4,000 children conceived by IVF and GIFT in the UK was reassuring. The overall incidence of malformations in these babies was no higher than in the country as a whole. However, even when the twins and higher multiple births were excluded, the babies were, on average, born slightly earlier than normal and were lighter by about 300 g.[2] The reason for the higher number of low birthweight and premature babies is not clear and needs further study. A partial explanation may be the higher rate of Caesarian section among these pregnancies, resulting in some babies being delivered earlier than they would have been otherwise.

Once the baby is born and seen to be healthy, most parents are enraptured and know that every painful stage passed on the way to this wonderful culmination has been worthwhile.

Others find their reaction may not be so straightforward. As friends and relatives rejoice for them, the parents may have times of doubt. Were those years of striving all for this – the sleepless nights, the chaotic house, the uncooked supper, a crying baby and an irritable, distracted partner? The problems are often compounded by the image of the competent, self-sacrificing, all-loving mother – or father – that grew over the long years of waiting.

At the MBF we have seen a number of despondent mothers in the Twins Clinic who have given up a high-powered job to devote themselves to full-time mothering and have been devastated by what they have seen as their failure. For women who have been responsible for running a large office, it is bound to be humiliating to feel incapable of coping with one home and only two small persons (and not least when a neighbour beautifully manages three under-fives on her own and without an A level, let alone a university degree). It is no wonder that several mothers have found that they, and the babies, become much happier when they return to work, particularly if this can be part time yet pays for the help they then need.

Development of the Children

But what of the outlook for the children resulting from IVF and DI? Are they likely to be as healthy and happy as those conceived spontaneously? What of their psychological development, and how do they relate to their parents?

Theoretically, psychological harm could come about in any of three ways: as a result of physical damage to the gametes or embryo; as a result of some sort of 'psychic' damage in the womb; or from emotional disturbance in the child when it – or other children – comes to learn about its unusual origins.

In practice any physical damage to a gamete or embryo

would probably have already resulted in the very early death of the embryo, if it was fully formed at all. The second idea, that of psychic damage in the womb, we find difficult even to comprehend, let alone believe. How could the fact in itself that the gametes were donated or fertilized in a dish have any such effect? After all, fertilization plainly happens well before the embryo develops any consciousness.

Psychological damage resulting from a child's learning about his or her unusual origins is clearly another matter, and has to be taken seriously. For a sensitive child to learn that his or her conception occurred in a laboratory dish could well be disturbing. Another child might be upset by learning that the (donated) egg or sperm came from someone he or she would never identify or meet.

On the other hand, some children could be equally unsettled to discover they were born out of wedlock, that they were fathered by someone else (a passing stranger), or that their mother had never really wanted children. None of these phenomena are unusual but a vulnerable child can be disturbed by all manner of things. Equally some children seem predisposed towards anxiety or depression but in general prove to be more robust than many people realize.

We may also recall that great numbers of children have learned that they were adopted – or 'specially chosen' – without appearing to suffer any noticeable harm. Artificially conceived children may similarly be told how much special effort was put into achieving their creation! They could be told Handel's reported response to the charge that, having been born in Germany, he was not a true Englishman: 'I am a better Englishman than you. You were born English. I *chose* to be English.'

The argument can only be resolved by producing empirical evidence, and fortunately the findings from the few studies undertaken so far are reassuring. A team at the Clinical and Health Psychology Research Centre of London's City University reported the results of a comparative study of over forty families in each of four groups. There were 41 who had had their children by IVF; 45 with a child conceived by donor insemination; and two control groups, one of 43 families with a child conceived naturally and one of 55 families with a child adopted in infancy. (The children in each group were between four and eight years old, with roughly equal numbers of boys and girls, and their parents were matched as closely as possible for age and social class.)

The quality of parenting and the presence of emotional and behavioural problems in the children were assessed by a standardized interview with each mother and questionnaires completed by both parents and the child's teacher. The children also underwent tests measuring their attachment to the parents, including both positive and negative feelings.

The results probably surprised those most anxious about potential psychological damage. If anything they suggest that the outcomes are better for children conceived by IVF or DI than for those conceived naturally. The quality of parenting in the IVF families was found to be superior to that of naturally conceiving parents, even when a donor had also been involved.

In terms of the children's emotions, behaviour or relationship with their parents, there were no significant differences between the groups. Regarding quality of parenting, those who conceived by means of IVF rated as well as adoptive parents. The authors concluded that genetic ties were less important for family functioning than the parents' strong desire for parenthood.[3]

Many people will have expected this finding. It is too easy to forget that many naturally conceiving parents may not have really wanted to have a baby. One or both may have had the child by mistake. By contrast both parents involved in assisted conception could hardly have acted more deliberately and have often spent many desperate years, and made great sacrifices, to secure their child's birth.

On the other hand, IVF mothers may find it particularly hard to combine motherhood with a job. Some Belgian psychologists found that overall there were no major differences in the quality of the parent–child relationship between IVF families and families with a naturally conceived child. However, they did find that IVF mothers who went out to work had more difficulty in their relationship with the child, showing less respect for the child's autonomy and less effectiveness in organization and limit setting compared with both non-working IVF mothers and working 'control' mothers. Having invested so much in the precious pregnancy, IVF mothers seemed to want more to stay at home with the child and felt guilty when they could not do so. The study also showed that their motives for returning to work were more likely to be financial, whereas those of naturally conceiving children mothers were more often those of personal development or to increase their social contacts.[4]

In Victoria, Australia, the growth and development of 314 IVF children were studied at the age of two and found to be similar to those of the general population. Again the quality of family relationships was, if anything, stronger among the IVF families. Yet, as we stress in Chapter 16, more and longer-term follow-up studies are needed.

The Enduring Infertility

To an outsider a pregnancy and the birth of a healthy child mark the end of a couple's infertility problem. For many couples this is true but some of the infertile say that, however many children they may have achieved, they not only remain infertile (which is technically true) but will never be rid of the pain of it. One woman, who had given birth to triplets following IVF, could identify the times when she felt like this. She wrote:

I go to the nursery school and two heavily pregnant women are comparing notes, from the physical side-effects of pregnancy to the colour of the wallpaper on the new nursery walls. I am excluded. It's not as if I have been through a second pregnancy so that I can join in their conversation. Being infertile is being excluded.

I know three people who are pregnant and don't want to be. They are angry: one has a good job and thought her family with three children was complete; another with four boys has just heard that it is another boy; the third who had a single baby and triplets by IVF has now conceived naturally. All have their reasons for being angry, but they have achieved a pregnancy. I feel angry with myself for not achieving a pregnancy. I suppose I have to learn to forgive myself.

I am continually asked, 'Are you going to have more children?' The answer is that I can't have children. Unlike others I don't have the choice.

This is how my infertility still invades my life. It is painful because it is a loss of ability on my part. In extreme it is the death of part of me and I suppose I am grieving about it. This all sounds crazy when I don't want to have more children. I just wish I could have had my children one at a time . . . I blame myself. I got myself into this situation because I was infertile. This is why I need to come to terms with my infertility despite being a mother of three.

Strictly speaking, a woman who has achieved a family through IVF has had her infertility not cured but circumvented, so the feelings of inadequacy can remain very real and should perhaps be discussed with a counsellor.

Others, however, readily put the painful journey behind them. Norma Chatel – writing in the *Prospect Newsletter* (March 1994) – described how over twenty years she had numerous doctors, a variety of drug treatments, three or four attempts at DI, five unsuccessful IVF treatments at one hospital and then, on the second attempt at another hospital, finally succeeded in having a daughter. At the age of forty-one she then had a second baby, having conceived spontaneously. She went on to say: 'The need to procreate is so fundamental I found it impossible to put it to the back of my mind. It was with me all the time – and now I am glad to say that it was because of my driving force that I finally delivered two beautiful daughters.'

8. Multiple Pregnancy

Throughout history twins have always been regarded as very special, and for many infertile couples the news that not one but two babies are on the way comes as a joyful bonus. Moreover this news of a ready-made family is becoming much more frequent. Many forms of infertility treatment substantially increase the chances of conceiving twins, triplets, quadruplets or even more.

Since they were first used in the 1960s, it was recognized that drugs that stimulate the ovaries to make more than one egg available for fertilization significantly increase the chances of a multiple birth. So does the common practice of placing two or three embryos in the womb during IVF treatment or eggs during GIFT. In the UK the transfer of more than three embryos into the womb is now illegal, but in some countries many more embryos have often been transferred with unfortunate results in terms of the vulnerability or mortality of the children and the strains upon their parents.

The multiple-pregnancy rate following IVF treatment is very high indeed. In 1992, 28.2 per cent of couples having babies had twins or more (compared with about 1.2 per cent in the general population). Of these 24.1 per cent were twins and 4 per cent triplets. For the first year since 1986 there were no IVF quads in 1991.

As we mentioned in Chapter 7, the number of embryos transferred during IVF treatment will influence the multiple-pregnancy rate. Of the pregnancies achieved following IVF in 1991 the percentage of multiple pregnancies was 32 per cent for three embryos; 26.2 per cent for two embryos; and 1.7 per cent for one. These last few multiple pregnancies, associated with the transfer of only a single embryo, are of course puzzling. They could have arisen either from a single zygote dividing to form identical twins or from a spontaneous conception which happened to occur at the same time, involving another egg which had escaped collection.

Some treatment centres are now, wisely, limiting the number of embryos transferred to two unless there are exceptional circumstances and certainly in younger patients.

Identical and Non-identical Twins

There are two types of twins: identical twins, otherwise known as monozygotic or uni-ovular; and non-identical twins, otherwise called dizygotic, fraternal or binovular.

Monozygotic twins arise when a fertilized egg, or zygote, splits into two during the first fourteen days after the egg has been fertilized. These two halves develop into separate individuals who have the same genetic make-up. Having the same chromosomes, the babies are bound to be of the same sex and to have very similar physical features. They may look quite different when they are first born if they have received unequal amounts of nourishment or been subjected to different physical pressures in the womb, but as they grow older they tend to look more alike. Their personalities may be quite different, however.

Dizygotic or non-identical twins result from two eggs that have been independently released in the same month and fertilized by two different sperm. Neither the genes nor, therefore, the looks of these twin children will be any more alike than those of any other brothers and sisters born to the same parents. In the UK about two sets of dizygotic twins are born for every monozygotic pair, although among those arising from treatment for infertility the proportion of dizygotic twins is considerably greater.

The Causes of Twinning

The causes of monozygotic twinning are still unknown and their incidence of about one in 300 pregnancies is the same throughout the world. (It has recently been noticed, though, that monozygotic twins occur slightly more often than expected following ovulation stimulation, whether given alone or as part of IVF. These cases may provide clues to the causes of monozygotic twinning in general.)

Although no single cause of dizygotic twinning is known, there are many associated factors, mostly related to the levels of gonadotrophins present in the mother. Factors affecting the twinning rate probably include genetic ones which come directly through the female line but may be carried by a father to his daughters. Race appears to have a strong influence, black races having a much higher rate than Caucasians and Asian Indians. The oriental ('Mongolian') races have the lowest rate.

The chance of having twins increases with the age of the mother, until her late thirties, and with her 'parity' or number of previous children. Tall women are more likely to have twins than short ones, and heavier women more likely than light.

Birth Rates for Twins

In the UK the twinning rate in 1992 was 80.5 per 1,000 pregnancies, which meant that about one in forty children was born a twin. Yet the number of twin conceptions is much higher than the number of twin babies actually born. One or both twins are often lost early in pregnancy, and before the advent of ultrasound scanning many of these twin pregnancies went unnoticed. Parents can have their hopes raised when two small sacs are seen on the first ultrasound scan, only to be dashed a few weeks later when one fails to develop.

This so-called 'vanishing-twin syndrome' is a particularly common if sad experience for couples receiving infertility treatment. They are more likely to have their first ultrasound scan very early in the pregnancy, whereas most pregnant women will not have theirs until one of the twin embryos has already disappeared.

Triplets and More

Theoretically there is no limit to the number of babies that can be produced at one delivery. In 1971 an Australian woman gave birth to nine babies (five boys and four girls). Two of the boys were stillborn; the remaining babies died within a week. The largest set with any survivors have been septuplets. The largest surviving complete sets are sextuplets. At least nine sets have been recorded worldwide, three of them in the UK (six girls in 1983, three boys and three girls in 1986 and one boy and five girls in 1993). All three of these sets were from mothers receiving infertility treatment.

The triplet rate in the UK used to be about one in 10,000 deliveries, but this figure has trebled since the introduction of hormone treatments and assisted conception. In 1992 the rate was one in 3,400 deliveries. Of infants born at over twenty-four weeks' gestation, there were 225 reported sets of triplets, 8 of quadruplets and 1 of quintuplets. In 1985–9 there were 47 sets of quads, compared with only 5 in 1965–9.

In some countries the number of triplet sets has increased even more dramatically than in the UK. There is an even greater increase in the number of surviving triplet children worldwide. Many of these very small babies would never have lived before the recent improvements in intensive care.

In spontaneously conceived triplets, according to calculations obtained from twin conceptions, about one-sixth of the sets should be of three identical children (monozygotic) and one-third should comprise an identical pair and one non-identical (dizygotic). The other half of the sets should consist of three non-identical (trizygotic) children. It turns out, however, that there is a somewhat higher incidence of dizygotic sets. Among assisted conceptions most, but not all, are trizygotic.

The Impact of Hormone Treatments

In the UK it is difficult to find out just how many twins result from different kinds of infertility treatment because many of the ovulation-stimulating drugs are prescribed by family doctors and are not centrally recorded. As we saw in Chapter 5, sometimes the drugs are given for quite different reasons and the recipients may be unaware that they are likely to make them more fertile, much less candidates for multiple pregnancy. Many have been shocked, some horrified. For instance, two mothers in the MBF's Supertwins Clinic had taken the drugs only to regulate their menstrual periods.

There is no doubt that all types of ovulation-stimulating drugs increase the chances of having a multiple pregnancy, some to a greater extent than others. In the East Flanders region of Belgium a careful record has been kept since 1976 of whether twin pregnancies are occurring spontaneously or are induced by treatment, and if so what sort. In seventeen years the number of doctor-induced twin pregnancies appears to have risen from 2 per cent of the total to 36 per cent. Of the 85 doctor-induced cases recorded in 1992, 51 were as a result of ovulation-stimulating drugs alone.[1] A British study of the use of Clomid in 2,369 pregnancies in 1981 found that 6.9 per cent resulted in twins. There were also eleven sets of triplets, seven of quads, and three of quins.[2]

Many couples appear to be told that their using Clomid entails no risk of conceiving triplets. This has certainly not been our experience. It may be that the potency of Clomid has been underestimated and many doctors have given too large a dose before the patient's response has been gauged.

Some other types of drug (see Chapter 5) are known to carry a still higher risk of multiple pregnancy, but this is now well recognized and responsible clinics are monitoring their patients closely. If there are signs that a woman is likely to produce a large number of eggs, she will be advised against having unprotected intercourse during that month. Unfortunately some hospitals still lack the equipment or discipline necessary to perform this monitoring, and at least one high multiple birth has been the result.

The only relevant British figures obtained so far were from a survey carried out in 1989, which found that approximately one-third of higher multiple births (that is, triplets or more) in that year had occurred spontaneously, a third following IVF or GIFT treatments and a third from the use of ovulation-inducing drugs alone.[3]

Similar figures have been reported from many other countries. Paul Lancaster reviewed the international results for 1989 and found figures for IVF twins ranging from 15 per cent in Germany to 26 per cent in the US, and for IVF triplets from 2 per cent in Australia to 6 per cent in France.[4]

A Shock Diagnosis

Even to those who have been warned of the risk, the diagnosis of a multiple pregnancy can come as a shock. Nor is the news always broken as sensitively or tactfully as it might. One mother's first indication that she was expecting quins was a flippant inquiry from the ultrasonographer as to whether she was good at knitting!

A multiple pregnancy with twins, let alone triplets, tends to be less comfortable than a single pregnancy, and many mothers will stop work earlier and require extra rest. In the case of triplets, particularly, many women will be admitted to hospital for rest during their pregnancy. Complications such as sickness, high blood pressure and premature labour are common.

Multiple pregnancies are much more variable in length than single ones, but on average twins will arrive at thirty-seven weeks, three weeks earlier than singletons; triplets three weeks earlier still. But many sets will be born much earlier. We have seen a set of triplets who were delivered fourteen weeks early, each weighing less than a kilogram, yet they all survived healthily.

Babies of Low Birthweight

The more babies delivered at one time, the smaller they are likely to be. They not only tend to be born earlier but have also competed for nourishment in the womb. The average birthweight of twins is 2.5 kg. (about 5.5 lb.), of triplets 1.8 kg. and of quads 1.4 kg., compared with an average weight for single babies of nearly 3.5 kg.

Those very small babies who survive do so at great cost to the neonatal services (as, sadly, do those who take time to die). The average cost in the UK of neonatal care for a triplet infant is 24 times that for a single baby and for a quad infant 42 times that for a singleton. This means that a quadruplet pregnancy costs 168 times that of a singleton pregnancy in terms of neonatal care alone.

The NHS bears the cost of the care of all such babies in Britain, even if the infertility treatment was provided by a private clinic. As the neonatal wards become increasingly over-crowded with such treatment-induced multiple births, many feel the cost should be borne by the clinics responsible for their conception or by their insurers.

These babies inevitably displace other sick babies from the neonatal units. If a hospital expects to deliver premature triplets, it may well have to close its neonatal intensive care unit to outside referrals of sick single babies, despite a lack of such facilities elsewhere. This can lead to intense resentment from the parents of the single babies and frustration for their doctors.

There is also the high cost of a pregnancy that includes longer hospital stays, more investigations such as ultrasound scans and frequently a Caesarian delivery.

Are They Identical?

Nearly all parents want to know whether the babies are identical or not, but far too many doctors wrongly think it is of little importance. We firmly believe that zygosity should be determined in all twin children at birth, and not only for the natural interest of the parents and later of the children themselves. It is also highly relevant to the clinical care of the babies, including the assessment of growth and development and to any genetic counselling that may be necessary later.

So how can zygosity be determined? A third of all sets of twins are boy/girl pairs and these must therefore be dizygotic. In like-sex twins, physical features are unreliable indicators at birth, but by two years of age one can usually tell just by looking at the children, particularly by scrutinizing their ear, feet and hand shape, teeth eruption and formation, and overall pattern of growth.

In about one-third of like-sex twins, the placenta is a helpful indicator. If it has a single chorion (outer sac) the twins must be monozygotic. However, one-third of monozygotic twins, as well as all dizygotic twins, have a dichorionic placenta (that is, with two outer sacs). A dichorionic placenta is *not*, therefore, a reliable indicator of dizygotic twins — despite the number of doctors and midwives who still believe it is!

In like-sexed twins with a dichorionic placenta, tests on

blood samples or the placenta are the only way to obtain a reasonably definite determination of zygosity. They can be tested for genetic markers such as blood groups, proteins and enzymes. The most accurate method is DNA testing on blood or the placenta, but this is expensive (and rarely provided within the NHS).

Life with Twins

For those who have had difficulty in becoming pregnant, the conception of twins is usually welcomed. Certainly twins offer many joys even if there is also a greater risk of medical, social and financial difficulties. Granted adequate help and support, most parents consider the advantages of having twins, and of being a twin, greatly outweigh the disadvantages.

Although most parents of triplets are devoted to them, most would say that this was not the best way to have children. It is not ideal for the children, their parents or any brothers and sisters. Departments of health and social services are also likely to be put under greater strain.

The Care of Triplets

Even when all three babies are strong and healthy, they are liable to put considerable stress on the family. As a result of a recent study of triplets conducted in the UK – in which Elizabeth Bryan participated – reliable information is, for the first time, available on the medical and social effects of triplets on families from the time of conception. This study looked at the lives of all British families who had triplets or more born in 1980–85 (excluding 1981) and many more families who had triplets born in 1985–8.[5]

The practical difficulties of looking after three babies at

the same time are plainly immense. No mother can even carry three babies at once. Only with the greatest difficulty can she feed or transport them by car, bus or train on her own. In practice many mothers do not take their babies out, so they become housebound. The consequent isolation, on top of the inevitable strain and tiredness, can easily lead to depression.

The study of triplets found that most families had inadequate help and such as they got often took prodigious efforts to procure. Relatives can rarely provide the necessary amount of dependable or predictable help, or are daunted by the responsibility of so many babies. It is not just tiring: there are too few hours in the day. A study by the Australian Multiple Births Association showed that it took 197.5 hours per week just to care for baby triplets and do the other necessary household tasks.[6] Unfortunately a week has only 168 hours.

It is sometimes assumed that most families with triplets must become rich from commercial sponsorship. But nowadays to get any useful funding you need at least five babies!

No couple asks for triplets yet many parents of triplets are distressed by the thoughtless or intrusive comments of friends, let alone strangers. Critical remarks are especially aimed at those whose babies result from infertility treatment. The implication is that the parents of triplets have 'asked for it' – a particularly cruel accusation for a couple who have been trying desperately for many years to have just one child.

The financial burden of triplets is plainly greater than that of three single children: clothes and equipment cannot be handed down from the eldest to the youngest child. Three high-chairs, three cots, three car seats and so on demand a punishing outlay, not to mention the larger home or car that most of them need. And all at once!

A previously working mother will also take much longer to get back to work and the father may be torn between working overtime to earn more money and spending more time at home to help with the babies. Feeding alone takes many hours.

There can also be problems for other children in the family. Being the brother or sister of triplets is an unenviable position. Not only is mother's time consumed by the care of the new arrivals but they get far more attention from relatives, friends and even passers-by. Life is especially hard for the toddler who was so recently the very centre of family life.

Special Support

As the number of children of higher multiple births continues to increase, their families must clearly be given the special support they need. Assistance from the health and social services has generally been inadequate and very patchy, yet the cost of greater investment would be handsomely recouped within only a few years in the form of healthier and less dependent families.

Parents of triplets welcome the opportunity to meet each other. Many such mothers have never met another set of triplets before, let alone talked to anyone with experiences of the practicalities of life with three babies at once. In Britain the Supertwins Group of the Twins and Multiple Births Association (TAMBA) will put parents in touch with each other (see Where to Find Help).

In addition, professional support for families with children of higher multiple births is offered by the MBF's Supertwins Clinic. Apart from seeing one of its paediatricians, families can lunch together and discuss each other's experiences. They will also learn from the parents who have volunteered to help (some of whose triplets are now adults) that the problems can be managed and that life really does improve for all concerned. Similarly, anxious expectant parents who have come for advance briefing are reassured to see so many healthy and happy babies.

Many of the problems presented by higher multiple births

can be surmounted, but some couples who are told to expect triplets, quads or more and fear the implications, may wish to consider a reduction of the pregnancy to, say, twins, in a procedure known as embryo reduction. Especially where there is a notably higher risk of miscarriage, or of disability or death of the children as a result of extreme prematurity, this highly problematic and controversial step may at least deserve discussion. Our next chapter treats this painful subject at some length, both for its own sake and as an example of the complex moral dilemmas attending the reproductive revolution in general.

9. Embryo Reduction of a Multiple Pregnancy: An Insoluble Dilemma?

Tragedies at birth often focus both medical and public attention on otherwise neglected problems. In 1985 Patti Frustachi of California gave birth to septuplets, allegedly as the result of following an ill-judged course of Pergonal (human menopausal gonadotrophin) and inadequate ultrasound monitoring. One septuplet was stillborn, three died over the following three weeks and the three survivors suffered impaired vision, hernias, chronic lung damage and developmental delay. A law suit, settled out of court in 1990, provided large payments to the Frustachis and monthly payments to the three survivors.[1]

Meanwhile, in 1987, Susan Halton gave birth in Liverpool to septuplets, all of whom died one after another, within sixteen days of their birth. The press closely followed this heartbreaking story and *New Society* called for the selective removal of some of the embryos in such high multiple pregnancies in order to enhance the chances of survival for the remainder.

Nearly ten years before, in 1978, a woman pregnant with twins went through a process known as selective fetocide, where the twin suffering from a severe metabolic disorder was killed in the womb. Such operations continued to be performed in cases of serious fetal abnormalities, but it was not until 1986 that a higher multiple pregnancy was reduced in number without abnormality being a factor. A letter to the *Lancet* then reported the reduction of a quintuplet pregnancy to twins and the birth of two healthy girls.

In the old days a couple faced with a multiple pregnancy of triplets, quadruplets or even more could only continue with the pregnancy, with all its attendant risks, or have a full termination. But after a long wait and years of infertility, to be left with not even one baby was especially cruel.

Now a third option is available, whereby the number of embryos is reduced by destroying one, two or more of them in the early weeks of pregnancy, so that two embryos (or sometimes three or just one) are left to develop normally. The procedure is known variously as embryo reduction (in the UK), multifetal reduction (in the US), fetal reduction, selective reduction or selective birth.

Confusion could arise here between the use of the terms 'embryo' and 'fetus'. According to embryologists, the embryo becomes a fetus after ten weeks' gestation. As reductions are usually performed somewhere between eight and twelve weeks of gestation, it may, strictly speaking, be either embryos or fetuses that are destroyed, so in this particular context the terms are generally used interchangeably.

Embryo reduction is a peculiarly difficult and painful subject, both emotionally and ethically, for medical staff as well as parents. It offers a choice which carries sadness either way. Yet the case for reduction can be a strong one, and many couples threatened with a high multiple pregnancy will at least want to consider the arguments before deciding what to do.

There are two extreme views. Those totally opposed to abortion are unlikely to approve of embryo reduction even though it is not aimed at stopping the entire pregnancy. At the other extreme are those who see it as wholly justified if it substantially improves the chances of producing one or two healthy babies instead of three or more who are all weak, handicapped or stillborn. In between there are people who have many hesitations about the procedure (including the possible long-term effects on the survivors), but who think it justified in some circumstances.

Parents should be counselled about the real possibility of a high multiple pregnancy before they even start infertility treatment, especially with hormones. (In Britain triplets may result from IVF or GIFT but rarely quads or more because the law limits the number of transferred embryos and eggs.) The option of embryo reduction should also be mentioned to couples well before they could be faced with such a choice. Too many couples hear about it only after their triplets or quads are diagnosed and are then horrified at an already stressful time.

Methods and Timing

There are various methods of destroying an unwanted embryo. One of the most common is an injection of potassium chloride into the embryo, which stops its heart. Another is aspiration (a sucking-out) of the sac containing the embryo. Both methods can be performed through the vagina or the wall of the abdomen. Whichever technique is employed, all the embryos remain in the womb, but the one, two or more that have died stop growing and are often absorbed. Any not absorbed do no harm to the remaining embryos.

Specialists differ about the best time to carry out an embryo reduction. Some advise doing it as early as 7–8 weeks; others suggest waiting until about eleven weeks. A balance must be struck between reducing emotional stress by getting the operation over quickly and allowing a few more weeks to detect a gross abnormality in any of the fetuses, which would make easier the choice of which embryos to be saved.

During the first ten weeks of a pregnancy one or more embryos may die in the womb, which is another reason for postponing the reduction. It is not uncommon to see, say, three sacs on the ultrasound scan at six weeks but a few weeks later just two sacs with growing fetuses and one small sac containing only the remnant of the third embryo. Later this sac may not be detectable at all.

Opting for Embryo Reduction

Many parents are especially and understandably distressed at the idea of having to choose which embryo should live and which should die. It is rarely possible, so early in the pregnancy, to 'select' the embryo, whether on grounds of freedom from abnormality, gender or anything else. 'Selective reduction' is therefore a misleading expression. True selection may become feasible as new techniques are developed, such as chorion-villous sampling, in which examination of placental tissue early in the pregnancy may detect abnormalities of the fetus. Meanwhile the accessibility of the embryos is the key – with a preference for leaving untouched the embryo (or embryos) nearest to the womb outlet. This, and sometimes the size of the embryo, is usually the basis for the necessary choice.

Deciding about an embryo reduction is bound to be diffi-cult for a couple and for their doctor. The risks and the balance of advantages and disadvantages will differ in each case, and the would-be mother and father may each have different thoughts and feelings about it. She may feel greatly distressed at disposing of a potential baby; he may no less shrink from the idea of one of his children being disabled. Partners are almost bound to disagree to at least some degree, so there must be a willingness to compromise as to what is best for them as individuals, as a couple and as a family.

It is worth rehearsing some of the arguments, for and against, which deserve careful exploration.

The Case for Embryo Reduction

For many couples the overriding aim will be the safe birth of the one healthy child they originally sought. Their next biggest concern may well be the health and welfare of any surviving twin or triplet.

Most triplets – perhaps quads – will end up as normal healthy children. Even a high multiple pregnancy can sometimes lead to the birth of entirely healthy children. There is, however, a distinctly greater risk of miscarriage or of low birthweight or very premature delivery with all the attendant complications. Disability in at least one of the children is therefore much more likely.

On the other hand, if the high multiple pregnancy is reduced to just one or two fetuses, there is a much greater chance of having a healthy baby (or twins) and greatly reducing the risk of some or all of them dying or being disabled. The chances of a tragic outcome increase if there are five or more fetuses. Some couples have to cope with their bereavement for the babies that did not survive as they face the difficult challenge of caring for both a disabled and a healthy child at the same time. In one set of quads conceived following GIFT, after twelve years of trying for a baby, the babies were born fourteen weeks early. One died after six days, the second after six months, having never left hospital. The third was severely disabled and the fourth a bright child but very small. The strain on that family was, understandably, enormous.

Unless a couple have wholly ruled out embryo reduction, their decision will broadly depend on the relative levels of risk of an adverse medical outcome, their attitudes towards the various stresses associated with higher multiple pregnancies and the possible consequences for their own situation and relationship. There is much honest debate in the medical profession and elsewhere both about the number of babies needed to justify a reduction and the appropriate number of embryos to leave. Opinions will be influenced by the doctor's own experience of the outcome of higher multiple pregnancies and of those pregnancies that have been reduced, and by the (so far few) reviews of such outcomes in the medical publications worldwide.

Unfortunately it is hard to make reliable comparisons because many treatment centres only report the outcome of pregnancies that have reached twenty, or even twenty-eight, weeks. The result is that the worst outcome – the loss of all the babies – often goes unreported. Yet according to a multi-centre study of 463 multiple pregnancies in which an embryo reduction had been performed, 84 per cent of the reduced pregnancies resulted in babies being delivered after twenty-four weeks (and therefore with a real chance of survival) and 84 per cent of these viable pregnancies were delivered after thirty-three weeks.[2]

Although twin pregnancies are recognized as somewhat riskier than single ones, most people with higher multiple pregnancies prefer a reduction to twins rather than to just a singleton. This is partly because the outlook for the survival of twins has greatly improved and partly because the couple may not have another chance to complete their family.

Occasionally parents expecting twins have asked their obstetrician to reduce the pregnancy to a single fetus, even where there are no medical grounds for it. Most obstetricians are very reluctant to do this and many refuse. However, the couple have sometimes then decided to take what they see as the only remaining alternative – a termination of the whole pregnancy. This must be the saddest outcome of all. Such situations pose painful ethical and human dilemmas for everyone concerned, and the distress of the medical staff themselves is often underestimated.

From the **medical** point of view most doctors would consider pregnancies with four or more embryos (and there has been a case with twelve) were at high risk and therefore that embryo reduction was a reasonable option where, of course, the parents wanted it.

In the case of pregnancies of three embryos, though, many

doctors would not now consider that there were strong medical reasons for a reduction, owing to recent improvements in the care and hence prospects of very sick premature babies. Other doctors would still recommend it, being partly – and understandably – influenced by the limited availability of neonatal intensive care locally.

For pregnancies involving four embryos or more, the question arises of whether to reduce the number to triplets or twins. As twins have a higher survival rate and tend to be born less prematurely than triplets, many doctors would recommend leaving two embryos rather than three. A recent study from Israel showed that in reducing either quad or quintuplet pregnancies, more babies survived as twins than as triplets, and were heavier and less premature at birth.

The Case against Embryo Reduction

There are several serious arguments against embryo reduction, and some less so. For example, taking the latter category, there is a slight risk of the procedure inducing a miscarriage of the whole pregnancy. But in most units this risk is smaller than that of miscarriage through continuing a pregnancy with three or more embryos. Other complications can result from the procedure, such as physical damage to the remaining embryos or the introduction of infection into the womb. Both are rare, however.

Some couples can hardly bear to contemplate destroying even part of a pregnancy, not least one they have striven so hard or long to achieve. Others may feel it is profoundly wrong to interfere so drastically with the processes of nature, or believe, indeed, that reduction amounts to a kind of murder.

Some couples may not have their own moral objections to the procedure but fear what their parents, family, friends or neighbours might say if word got out about what they had done. Some worry about their family doctor's reaction. Embryo reduction is, after all, such a recent medical development that many doctors, let alone would-be parents, have hardly heard of it, least of all got their minds round it. And with so novel a procedure, many instinctively decide not to go through with it, even though the case for it may seem objectively quite reasonable.

Some couples, for moral or religious reasons, would refuse outright to consider an embryo reduction under any circumstances. Others would consider either a termination of pregnancy or an embryo reduction only if an embryo (or fetus) was abnormal and never where potentially healthy babies were involved. Yet others believe choosing between embryos is in itself too arbitrary to be morally tolerable. Many couples doubt whether they could themselves handle such emotional confusions arising from so unusual a procedure. As one woman put it: 'How could you choose him but not her? What would I say to the survivor? That it was like a lucky dip?'

What, if anything, will eventually be told to the child is a very important question. Could it harm the child to learn that he or she could so easily have been terminated in the womb and that his or her siblings had been killed at the parents' request? Or will it be kept secret? Can such attempted secrecy itself cause harm in the family?

The question also arises as to whether damage of a more subtle, 'psychic' nature could be caused to the survivors. There is some evidence that the surviving child of a twin pregnancy may be aware of having been a twin. If this is so, the idea of damage to survivors of a higher multiple pregnancy is not inconceivable. We ourselves doubt the hypothesis but there is as yet no hard evidence either way.

Views in the Profession

One American study interestingly suggests that some medical professionals and lay people who would not object to a termination of a singleton pregnancy would refuse to contemplate the selective reduction of a higher multiple pregnancy through fear of it damaging the remaining embryos. In reality, the overall risk to the babies is greater if the higher multiple pregnancy continues than if it is reduced to twins.[3]

Assumptions about the mother's intentions may have been a factor here. An abortion is carried out because the mother, for often complex and varied reasons, does not want a child or feels unable to look after it. In contrast a mother who finds herself with a higher multiple pregnancy may seek an embryo reduction precisely because she desperately wants the best possible chance of a healthy child.

The American study also indicated that medical staff with the greatest knowledge of the complications of higher multiple pregnancy, such as specialists and geneticists in fetal medicine, were more accepting of embryo reduction than their colleagues. The degree of acceptance also varied according to religious group (Roman Catholics being the least accepting); depth of religious conviction; and nationality (Americans tending to be more accepting). Some of the people interviewed, however, believed abortion was unacceptable but that embryo reduction could be ethically justified when the higher multiple pregnancy carried a significant risk for either the fetuses or the mother, and where this risk could thereby be reduced.

The Law on Selective Reduction

Until a few years ago many obstetricians in the UK would not perform embryo reductions out of fear of legal action, and the perverse consequence was that some couples felt forced to proceed to a total termination. The legal situation regarding embryo reduction then changed with the introduction of the HFE Act of 1990, which rewrote part of the 1967 Abortion

Act. This makes it clear that embryo reduction, like abortion, may be carried out lawfully in defined circumstances.

Most reductions of higher multiple pregnancies will be legally justifiable on the grounds of substantial risk (due to premature birth) of the baby being born with 'such physical or mental abnormalities as to be seriously handicapped'. Risks to the mother's health alone will often justify reduction. These include excessive vomiting, high blood pressure, polyhydramnios (excess fluid in the womb), placental bleeding and pulmonary embolism.

The Outlook

How is a couple who opts for an embryo reduction going to feel about it in years to come? This is difficult to predict: the procedure has not been available for very long. Judging from our discussions at the Multiple Births Foundation with parents who have had their pregnancy reduced, most seem to feel later that they had made the best decision. Nevertheless some of them do feel sad and even guilty about losing babies that might otherwise have gone on to become healthy children.

And what about the effects on the surviving children? Whether embryo reduction has any particular consequences for the physical or emotional development of the surviving children is not known, as no follow-up studies have yet been completed. So far, though, the children appear to be developing quite normally.

For some couples the very suggestion of an embryo reduction is abhorrent. One couple said they could not have contemplated such an action even after they had lost their four little boys, one after the other. The mother has agreed to our quoting what she wrote about her visit to her obstetrician, having just heard she was expecting quads.

Before he had a chance to say anything, we told him that we had decided to keep all our babies. We knew there were risks, but I felt so special, quads are so very rare. It was like I had been chosen to have these children: even though I had only known them for a few days, I loved them so very much. I had plans for them . . . He told us that he hoped one baby would abort itself so that the others had a much better chance of survival. I was horrified – I know why he said it and I truly respect his reasons, but it doesn't alter the fact that it hurt so very much.

We have known some couples who decided not to have their quads reduced but have bitterly regretted this when the pregnancy ended in death and disability for one or more of the babies. On the other hand, one mother who chose to continue with a quintuplet pregnancy still felt she had made the right decision despite losing four sons and being left with one very frail daughter.

The MBF publishes a helpful leaflet on the subject and can give more personal advice about dilemmas that are bound to be difficult and painful, and are indeed ultimately insoluble. The would-be parents can only do their best when new but sad choices prove inescapable.

10. **Adoption as an Alternative**

After infertility treatment has failed or proved impracticable, the couple will naturally think of adoption as their only remaining chance of having a family. But as we shall see, adoption is neither easy to achieve nor the only option.

Some couples will try their utmost to adopt a healthy baby, but in many countries, including Britain, there are now very few available for adoption. Some couples may be prepared to adopt a baby from abroad, perhaps from a developing country. Some may wish to adopt a baby or child with mental or physical disabilities or other special needs. Such children are much more readily available. About 17,000 of the children in the care of local authorities in England and Wales could be placed for adoption if willing couples, individuals or families could be found.

Another option is fostering or custodianship – a longer-term form of fostering which gives parents more day-to-day rights. Another response, of course, is for the infertile couple to accept their childlessness and, as described in the next chapter, draw such satisfaction as they can from other sources.

All the options are attended by their own difficulties, and some general points should first be made about adoption, a particularly sensitive and controversial subject.

In Britain a couple who have finally decided to give up trying for their own baby and consider adopting someone else's will need to apply to their local social services department or an officially registered adoption agency (a list of addresses is published by the British Agencies for Adoption and Fostering: see Where to Find Help). But they will need to recognize that they are likely to be beginning another long and demanding process while in an already emotionally strained state. When infertility treatment eventually proves fruitless, the reaction of one or both of them may be to rush out at once to acquire a baby in order to staunch the grief.

Under these circumstances they will not succeed, and rightly. The first principle of adoption is that it is for the benefit of the child, not of the would-be parents. The child's needs have to be paramount. In most Western countries, at least, the public bodies and charitable agencies who place babies or children for adoption will take quite some time assessing the candidates and will rule out any whom they think are still emotionally disturbed, however understandably, by their experience of infertility treatment. Even after they are accepted, would-be parents may have to wait for up to two years before they get a baby.

In most European countries very few healthy babies are now offered for adoption. This is because contraception is much more effective and widespread than it used to be and abortion is now both legal and widely available. And, fortunately, far fewer unmarried women are shamed into giving up their babies than they were only a few decades ago. As a result, for every healthy baby there is a queue of potential parents, and the adoption agencies can afford to be highly selective. The infertile couple therefore need to think long and hard before risking yet more disappointment.

Legally speaking, adoption is as definite and total a commitment as genetic parenthood. The adopting couple become the legal parents. The child takes their name and will inherit from them just as if they had given him or her birth. Arguably the parents' responsibility for the adopted child is greater than for a natural child since they have deliberately taken on the responsibility by solemn and formal commitment. One's own child may not be planned: an adopted one certainly is.

Interviewing the Couple

The would-be adopters (or indeed foster parents) should question their motives very carefully before embarking upon adoption. Any social worker pursuing the best interests of the child will ask both members of the couple, together and separately, many questions that could seem intrusive, even impertinent.

First of all, he or she may ask whether the couple have thoroughly worked through the grief at failing to have their own children. Have they accepted help with this? Is their desire to adopt a child a calmly measured one, taking account of all the difficulties involved? Is the decision fully shared by both partners? Can they both stand up to close interviewing about it? Can they each acknowledge their own strengths and weaknesses and deal together and constructively with issues where their ideas conflict?

If they are adopting an older child, are they prepared to stop seeking infertility treatment and even use contraception rather than risk producing their own child after all, thereby precipitating what could well be a new crisis for a child who has probably already suffered undue upheaval in its life? (Some agencies will expect couples to act similarly even if it is a baby they are adopting.)

Many other questions will be asked. Have the interests of any existing children been fully considered and, if old enough, may they too be questioned? How much support does the wider family offer, or friends? How adaptable are the couple? If they have had years of childlessness, however reluctantly, have they settled into a lifestyle that has become too rigid or comfortable to absorb the continuing commotions and strains of parenthood? Will they remain patient and resolute? Might their adopted child always be thought of as somehow second best?

Some of the questions are especially hard. How stable is the partnership? To what extent can it cope with unpredicted stresses? Can the couple discuss impending moves, possible job changes, sexual difficulties? Is one of them a well-read know-all, yet who lacks a capacity for feeling and real responsiveness? Is the other one perhaps too independent, unready either to acknowledge his or her failings or to accept help?

And so it may go on. How well does each partner really know the other, or him- or herself? Has their sense of humour survived their emotional trials, and can they still laugh at themselves? Even after an interview like this?!

Many of these questions (though not all of them) are taken from a booklet offered by PPIAS, the Parent to Parent Information on Adoption Services (see Where to Find Help), and they wisely add: 'Don't panic if you can't answer all these questions confidently. We are all human and children need parents not paragons!'

Qualifications for Adoption

Infertile couples will generally be given priority, but most adoption agencies will insist not only that diagnosis and treatment should have finished but that the couple have come to terms with this. Some require a year's, or even two years', gap from the end of infertility treatment and the start of the assessment. Couples stand a better chance if they have already adopted one baby.

Most adoption agencies expect couples not only to be married but to have been together for at least three years. However, they may hesitate about a married couple who have been childless for ten or fifteen years and might have become set in their ways.

Age is a cruel handicap for many of the infertile who want to adopt a young baby. Out of concern for the long-term future of the child, many agencies rule that the wife should be under thirty-five and the husband under forty. Yet many of the infertile will have tried to start a family late and then used up more precious years on ultimately fruitless attempts. Many in Britain believe this rigidity should be removed, recognizing that people in their forties have much to contribute in the care and upbringing of adopted children.

We ourselves were barred from adopting a baby on grounds of age. Many agencies also dislike any great age difference between the couple. They will not expect the would-be parents to be well off, but they will ask about their financial position and how secure it is.

Adopting Babies from Abroad

It is so difficult to find a healthy British baby to adopt that many consider seeking one from abroad. Some positively like the idea of taking on a child from one of the less-developed countries and we know couples who have done this very successfully. It is, however, a complex issue. Most developing countries would prefer richer nations to give aid on the spot rather than take their children away. Nor do they always have proper adoption regulations and controls, and this has aroused fears of abuse of the system, where illegal smuggling, profiteering or even abduction may be involved.

As a result a Hague Convention on inter-country adoption was concluded in 1993 and Britain, like other countries, is expected to implement the new framework that has been created. So far as we know, no British adoption agency will bring babies from abroad, and parents hoping to make their own arrangements should be aware that they need to be as carefully screened as those adopting British children. The BAAF or the PPIAS may be prepared to offer advice but are likely to warn about both the practical and the ethical complications.

Useful contacts may also be made through STORK, the association for families who have adopted children from abroad (see Where to Find Help).

Issues of Race

In questions of adoption,, racial issues are especially complex and sensitive. In the UK proportionately more black than white babies become available, and in the past many black children were placed with wholly white families without much controversy. But in recent decades British opinion, echoed by agency practice, has increasingly sought ethnic and cultural compatibility between the adopted child and its new parents. There is much to be said for this, especially when a black child in a white family first meets varieties of prejudice and hurt that his or her white adoptive parents cannot themselves have experienced.

Yet we have known several successful adoptions of black children by white parents and sympathize with the 'Children First' campaigners who say the first priority is that every child needing parents is enabled to secure them, whatever their colour. This view takes on extra relevance in that many members of Britain's Asian communities seem reluctant to adopt Asian children where little (or 'too much') is known of their parents. Nor are black adoptive parents always easy to find.

There have been several much publicized cases where couples of mixed race have been refused adoption because they had allegedly had too little experience of racial abuse. (A Norfolk adoption panel called one couple 'racially naive'.) The British White Paper of 1993 therefore proposed that ethnic background should not be the ultimate deciding factor and that a general view of the couple's suitability should be made in each case. Such flexibility would surely be welcome.

Children with Special Needs

Nowhere is the need for loving parents greater than among children who have suffered the emotional damage of neglect, rejection, abuse or interrupted or indifferent care from their own parents, foster parents or from their children's homes or other 'caring' agencies. Many such children are physically healthy but have had difficulty in making close bonds with adults or in continuing to trust them after troubles or new disappointments arise. Sometimes their behaviour is erratic or worse. Moreover some of the children understandably want to be adopted together with one or more of their siblings. Apart from the family ties, these may have provided their only continuous relationships. Ideally, of course, siblings would be adopted together, but this is not always easy to achieve in practice.

Children with mental or physical disabilities are another needy group whose care and nurturing can be very rewarding. Such children would include those with Down's syndrome, cerebral palsy and spina bifida. Many of these children – other than those with Down's syndrome – will be of normal intelligence. All of them need love and all will repay love.

We are speaking here of several different categories of children, and further generalization would be treacherous at best. But it has to be said that the depth of the would-be adopters' compassion is an inadequate guide to their capacity to take on the child in question.

We ourselves carefully considered applying for an older child but had finally to admit that we really wanted a baby. We did not feel guilty about this. As two professional people with somewhat hectic and necessarily mobile lifestyles, we knew that, with some outside help, we would cope more easily with a baby than with a possibly demanding child whose need for attention and affection might well be prodigious. A successful adoption marries up the needs and capabilities of the child and the new parents. We had to recognize that most of our own needs for a child were essentially for a baby. Nor would we risk yet another emotional disaster befalling a child who had already suffered quite enough.

The Procedures for Adoption

If a couple choose adoption, they should apply to their Local Authority's adoption agency and other charitable agencies in their area, giving details about themselves and the kind of child they are looking for. Many agencies say their waiting list is full. But if one of the partners belongs to an ethnic or religious minority, the couple's chances of gaining an agency's interest may be greater, so it is worth giving such details.

Some agencies concentrate on placing children with special needs, and BAAF acts as a central exchange for many of these. It also provides helpful leaflets which potential adopters would be wise to read, together with books on the subject, before making a definite application.

The agency may suggest that would-be parents attend a 'preparation meeting' to talk with existing parents of adopted children and other candidates. If not previously warned by their family doctor or someone else, some couples may be upset to hear how few babies may be found for adoption or to learn about the sometimes distressing background of the children who are available to be adopted. (The press 'advertisements' for these older children cannot always tell the full story, for understandable reasons of confidentiality.) If all goes well, though, the agency will agree to arrange for a social worker to interview the couple in depth during a 'home-assessment programme'.

An agency's expenses are large and its staff time is valuable, so once a couple have got this far they are not expected to contact other agencies unless they become interested in a particular 'advertised' child. In that case they should at once say so. If the couple are selected, a suitable child will eventually be found, although this often takes time. If the child has special needs, the couple will receive not only full details of the child's condition and medical advice but appropriate counselling well before the procedure is completed.

In Britain a number of changes in procedure and philosophy were foreshadowed in the 1993 White Paper. Assuming the expected legislation is passed, children over the age of eleven will have the right to decide whether an adoption should go ahead and to take part in their own adoption hearing with their own legal representation. The Bill will also require courts, local authorities and adoption agencies to consider a child's welfare into adulthood. Rejected couples will have a complaints procedure.

This is not the place to describe how the couple go to court for an adoption order, or to give details about their legal rights and those of the natural parents after the order is granted. Nor have we space to go into what the process might cost, what prior medical examinations are necessary, nor what happens if the adoption goes wrong, or actually fails. There are many books on the subject, and BAAF and PPIAS, among others, will be pleased to give advice. ISSUE would also advise about counselling for those who suffer further disappointments by failing to adopt a child.

Fostering

If the infertile couple decide not to adopt or are told they are unsuitable, how likely is it that fostering would satisfy their needs?

Fostering is the formally approved (and subsidized) care of someone else's child for a period that may last several weeks, months or years. The fostered child is in no sense the couple's own child and never becomes this. For good or ill, the arrangement is intrinsically temporary. For this reason alone, fostering is unlikely to satisfy the infertile couple's desire for a family. Indeed they would be in danger of a new form of bereavement when the baby or child moves on. The longer the fostering lasts, and the more the child is loved, the more painful the eventual separation will be.

A possible exception is that represented by custodianship, a relatively recent legal innovation in the UK, whereby those who have fostered a child for some time can be granted more day-to-day rights than foster parents would normally be entitled to. However, they cannot change the child's surname and, in any legal sense, the relationship ends when the child reaches eighteen. Local social services departments will explain this in more detail, including the new 'foster-plus' status mentioned in the 1993 White Paper, which is meant to give long-term foster parents extra security.

It is, of course, easier to become a foster parent, or custodian, than an adoptive parent. But in practice most fostering agencies would probably hesitate to choose an infertile couple unless the couple had previous experience of rearing a child, whether their own or someone else's. An agency would not only want evidence of parental competence; it would be anxious that the couple might invest too much emotion in their relationship with the child and therefore make it more difficult for the child eventually to move on.

If adoption proves impossible, and if fostering is unlikely to satisfy the infertile couple, what options remain? Here we turn to childlessness: the processes of accepting and becoming reconciled to that state.

11. The Family That Never Was: Coping with Childlessness

A stranger who wandered round our house and was then told we had no children would be baffled. Our largest bedroom is full of toys, including a large doll's house, fifty or more dolls from all over the world, children's furniture, children's games, model cars. There is even a cradle. Everything is there, from fluffy dogs for tiny tots to books for studious teenagers. Half hidden by shrubs at the end of the lawn nestles a home-made children's house, also filled with toys, and a sand pit too often clogged with leaves.

Our visitor might think we had once had children but had lost them and now live mournfully in a sort of museum, or that we had never had children but live in a permanent fantasy. Both are disturbing images. This couple in their half-timbered house on a hill above the Golden Valley might seem to be locked either into a monument to unresolved bereavement or an illusion of perpetual play with children who never breathed. There, across the valley, the Black Mountains of Wales fade into lovely distance while here lies a seemingly blacker hole of concealed despair.

The truth is quite different. Yes, we wanted children passionately and we both suffered in our long search for them. Sometimes we still dream about them, still feel the old hurts. Yet, despite all this, we are not only reconciled to being without a family but sometimes delight in the sense of freedom and opportunity this deprivation has eventually allowed us.

Why, then, all the toys? Most of them date from Libby's youth and have accompanied her in her decades of work with children. Nothing gives her greater joy than their joy and their responsiveness. But why did Ronald build the garden house? Because he too enjoys children – if in more limited numbers and less frequently – and their ability to bring out the clown in him. For both of us a child can reach parts that no other human can reach.

Fortunately we can often have children to stay. Libby's two sisters have five young ones between them. Some of our twenty godchildren are now producing offspring. Friends often bring their young to this house and garden so enticingly equipped with treasure troves, hiding places and every form of entertainment.

We hope we have got the balance about right, for us: an enduring sense of loss counterbalanced by substantial measures of distraction, compensation and opportunities gladly seized. No one pattern will suit everyone, but we do think all these elements have some part to play. Our own balance took years to reach and we sometimes have relapses of one kind or another. We certainly had to go through all the fraught and wearing stages of bereavement before recognizing, let alone enjoying, any of the positive sides of childlessness.

The Stages of Grief

The final recognition that one will never ever have a family can feel like a profound bereavement. (The frustration of a couple's desire for a second child may sometimes be nearly as painful as failing to have a first.) For most people an initial numbing shock is followed by denial (that the loss has actually occurred); anger; envy; resentment; and sometimes guilt. There is usually a period in which they work through all these feelings, until they reach the final stage of gradual acceptance of their condition.

The different stages of this process may be short or long. They may overlap and will vary in their degree of prominence.

Not everyone will go through all stages nor feel them as deeply. What is important is that each individual goes through the different stages of grieving at her or his own pace. Friends and relatives may encourage one to get over it more quickly, partly out of care but partly for their own sake. The partner may take the same line. This is almost always misguided advice. Each of us can only move at our own speed, ideally without added pressure or guilt.

Many of the bereaved do not even recognize their feelings – for example, their anger with their partner, the doctors or with God. They may think this emotion unseemly, irrational, somehow inadmissible. Others project their anger on to other people, passionately resenting those who have had an abortion, who mistreat their children or just take having a family for granted.

The initial emotions may be so impossibly strong that they almost paralyse the sufferer. Some people can no longer drive a car, shop sensibly or choose a newspaper. Others feel lost, empty, bleak, overwhelmed. Some cannot sleep; some can only sleep. Many come close to driving their partner to despair.

Others may experience overwhelming feelings of guilt about a previous abortion or infection. And others may refuse to acknowledge these feelings because they are unbearable or irrational. In most people they are indeed irrational. But if the guilt is felt, it deserves attention, respect and, of course, eventual remedy.

Sometimes the deprived couples may simply not identify their childlessness as a form of bereavement. Some secretly carry on hoping against all the odds, if only to postpone the inevitable pain and misery of giving up hope.

Initial Shock

Many couples will suffer a severe sense of shock when they finally realize they will never have a child. The shock may arise as a result of a medical verdict, an inability to pay for yet another course of IVF or being unexpectedly refused a child for adoption.

At this time it is critical for the partners to cling together as best they are able and get what help they can through the family doctor or a local support group. They should not worry whether their reactions are normal, 'excessive' or different from each other's. 'Clinging together' may be especially hard at this most difficult time. Some couples may never have found this easy: one or both partners may resent over-dependency or fear it. Some do not have a sufficiently strong or rich partnership, or may already have felt cracks opening up. There may be blame, contempt, guilt or anger.

We each react very differently. The most sensible response may be to experience the terrible feelings for what they are, but at the same time to try to keep going, and keep together, until the bereavement can be coped with in a more gradual fashion. This may not always be possible. Each partner grieves in his or her own, sometimes very different, way, and mutual blame, rage, even hate, may tear a couple apart.

Depression

Whether or not the final verdict comes as a surprise, one or other partner is likely to feel very low, and there is bound to be some danger of a depression which will impair the couple's capacity to work or even function adequately. If this happens, professional advice is certainly needed. Otherwise this dreadful period just has to be lived through; shared where possible, sometimes just endured.

Depression is not uncommon following failed attempts at IVF, and anyone especially prone should seek help before it settles in. Unfortunately the depressed often don't believe that help is possible and don't even give it a chance. Whatever else they do, neither partner should listen to those clumsy commands to 'pull themselves together'. Such instructions are callous over-simplifications and when they inhibit mourning are potentially damaging to the future psychological health of the sufferer. Nor does it help if the adviser says he or she knows just how the victim feels! Ostentatious courage in the face of adversity may suit the hero, heroine or puritan, but will at best preserve only outward composure. The larger courage acknowledges and stays with the actual feelings, however they develop.

The Importance of Expressing Grief

For many infertile couples the possibility, even likelihood, of failing to have children will have been present throughout. As in our own case, each failure of a treatment brought frustration and distress but no sudden shock. When we finally decided to stop trying, it was partly because we had tried almost everything, but more because Elizabeth could no longer bear the awful oscillation between hope and despair. Hope can be cruelly painful. For many people the uncertainty is the hardest of all; the emotional see-saw is deeply wearing.

The grief was real for us both, though especially for her. In the end she knew there remained no realistic hope, yet could hardly believe we should never have children of our own. Even when childlessness has been essentially accepted in theory, it is not easy for a woman, or sometimes her partner, to resist the seductive whisper of 'miracles can happen', until yet another menstrual period comes round. Deciding to give up trying is one thing: giving up hoping is quite another. A visceral hope can persist even when all reasoned hope has been abandoned.

We did not hesitate to talk the experience through with our closest friends, though we did try, sometimes unsuccessfully, to avoid upsetting or boring them. Elizabeth dreamed constantly of embryos. After a year or so we went away for an experiential weekend on 'personal growth' and she spent hours in a corner of the studio painting them. She kept the images rolled up behind the wardrobe for years afterwards – an outward but deeply private expression of a profound inner experience, especially of our one pregnancy that had so sadly ended after ten weeks.

We tried many ways of working through our grief, not least creatively – of bodying it forth in some fashion, however artistically lame the result. We hoped that exploring our sense of loss would stop our feelings becoming repressed or clogged up. In our case we mostly used the written word to express ourselves, but sometimes drew, moulded clay or made pots. In addition Ronald had his poultry and their families. Once he hatched a deserted guinea fowl's egg under his armpit and reared the little bird for weeks afterwards, partly in a waste-paper basket placed between us in bed. He also propagated even more house plants than usual.

Writing about the experience, whether in a notebook, diary or as a story, can be a great help and can be done entirely in private. It does not matter if the results are literate, let alone literary. No one else need ever see it. But getting the story down on paper – or perhaps tape – can be surprisingly illuminating and therapeutic: we often do not know what we think or feel until we write it down or talk about it.

Unexpressed feelings can cause friction between partners. Frustrated hopes can lead to aggressive blame, and the partner often takes the brunt. Failure to share grief openly can cause misunderstanding and resentment. This is especially likely where one partner, denying his or her own feelings, suggests the other's grief is becoming excessive or morbid. (Which is not to deny that ultimately it can prove to be so.)

Alternatively the unexpressed grief may accumulate and fester in the unconscious until, perhaps many months or even years later, it erupts in unexpected and distressing forms. One woman told us sadly how she had lost a precious friendship just when she needed it most. A year after this woman had suffered an early miscarriage following infertility treatment (about which she had told no one), her best friend had her first baby. The woman found herself quite unable to visit her and, even worse, felt unable to explain this to her. Naturally the friend felt hurt and alienated.

Bottled-up grief can act like delayed shock and catch both partners unaware. Men may be especially prone to this: we have known some who were shattered by the experience, not least because they had long ignored or neglected their feelings.

To return to our own experience: when we wanted to cry or shout or to talk endlessly, we simply did so. If either of us had remained buttoned up, we hope we would have sought personal or professional advice of some kind. A counsellor can often help an inhibited partner to face up to his or her feelings.

Just as we sometimes do not know what we think until we say it, we may not know how we feel until we have expressed it. And what is there to lose? Other people will often know what we are going through even though we remain stolidly silent. And to watch someone struggling to keep control can be more painful for friends or colleagues than watching them cry. The novelist E. M. Forster warned that undemonstrativeness could eventually reduce the very capacity for feeling itself. Feelings cannot develop or flourish when they remain so diligently unexpressed, and the whole person can become psychologically impoverished as a result.

Think, by contrast, of those televised scenes of the bereaved crying out, tearing at their clothes, embracing their dead, in the Bosnian war, the Somali conflict, the Lebanon and Rwanda. These people do not lack dignity: they express their grief frankly, fully and unapologetically. They let it shake them, body and soul. They throw their arms round each other. Grief unites, not separates them, and does its necessary work. The bereaved then learn more swiftly how to live with and move on beyond their loss.

As we have suggested, if someone wants to cry out with pain, anger or grief, they should do just that. There is no right or wrong response when facing the extremities of life, so long as we avoid losing all control and needlessly distressing others. Nor should anyone feel guilty when they suddenly laugh again, have a good meal, go to a party. There will still be times of tears as well as times of apparent forgetfulness.

Partners in Grief

Much of what we have said has been in rather general terms but many more practical suggestions can be made and we are indebted to Diane and Peter Houghton's book *Coping with Childlessness*,[1] based on their long experience with ISSUE – at that time the National Association for the Childless (NAC).

Once it is clear that there will not be children, a couple will ideally stop worrying about the causes, let alone whose 'fault' the failure might be. This is much easier said than done but is probably crucial. What can be hardest of all is avoiding that dreadful internal refrain of 'If only . . . (we had done so and so)'. Neither partner should go on feeling guilty about the failings of their body or their past life. Such guilt is usually pointless, even destructive, but in men particularly it may be powerfully felt. For many men the loss of their fertility, the conclusion of their genetic line, may cause their most intense feelings of bereavement, whereas to the woman what is at the root of her grief is the loss of the baby that never was.

Men often suffer psycho-sexual problems on hearing of their infertility. Moreover, when there is no longer hope of a pregnancy, his partner, feeling that sex has cheated them or lost its purpose, may unwittingly collude by no longer encouraging love-making. Resuming a normal spontaneous sex life after many years of diary-dictated performance may take a long time. Both partners will need to be gentle with themselves let alone each other.

The couple will need to decide how much they will say, and to whom, about their final disappointment. There are usually some people who have to be confided in soon, such as relatives. It may be wise to take this rather slowly, but one or two people may need to be told straight away because they are likely to find out in any case or will be unduly upset if they only discover by accident or at second hand.

The couple need to agree upon their story (ideally it should be true, and short!) and how much to say to whom. We told our story plain and straight, if only to curb speculation (and the desperate business of trying to remember to whom we had not told what). Many years later we still reply, 'Sadly not', when asked the standard social question, 'Do you have children?' The questioner does not then feel obliged to ask any more questions and is spared accidentally making a tactless remark. We also feel we should do our small bit to help make infertility a less taboo-ridden subject.

Nevertheless we try not to overburden our friends with the subject, and still sometimes fail. To share your pain with those close to you is right, but not to harp on about it. Friends may need the time to impart their own troubles, after all.

No Cure for Grief

We must not pretend to have found a cure for grief. There may for many years be spurts of envy, frustration or pain, and surges of anger against whomever or whatever is held responsible. Many lose their faith for a while. Others feel angry with a God who has failed to give them what they most want in life. In the words of one of our correspondents: 'What makes this sort of bereavement difficult and protracted is that it is a loss of one's future, rather than one's past (as with the death of people one loves). There is an aspect of the bereavement that is never really finished with: we can expect to feel the pain of loss many times over in the future.'

For many years Elizabeth continued to have dreams of labour, giving birth and breastfeeding. Ronald still cries when reading letters from the infertile.

Many years after one woman had 'got over' not having children, she burst into what she called 'absurd' tears when Prince Edward was born. Others have found the birth of a friend's first grandchild unexpectedly upsetting. Some of the childless have found it hard to talk with those who have lost a real child, rather than a pregnancy or the hope of one, being envious of those with tangible memories to cherish. Bereaved parents at least enjoy recollections of the lost one and have greater public recognition of their pain, while the bereavement of the childless is often denied. No one has actually died. There has been no ceremony, no funeral.

The sense of bereavement lasts a very long time – perhaps, for some, a lifetime. And being childless can set a woman apart: the great and enviable world of mothers and their children excludes them. She may feel isolated: while she is at work she may think of her neighbours happily exchanging experiences of parenthood at toddler groups, or sharing hints about child management at the school gate.

It is sometimes harder for a childless couple to feel part of their own extended families. They may feel excluded, albeit unintentionally. Family get-togethers are often centred on one of the children – a christening, coming of age or wedding. Christmas can be especially difficult, and it is unlikely that the childless couple's home will be where the family gathers.

Some people react emotionally to what is perhaps too often called 'failure' to have children. They may feel shame and humiliation but also a loss of drive or ambition. When there is no one special to hand the baton of life on to, people can ask, what is all the effort worth?

The answer has to be, a very great deal: life itself, with all its wonders, to be shared by ourselves and by others. Although the childless are bound to continue grieving, it is vital for them to become open again – to all forms of distraction, compensation and opportunity.

Distraction

Even within a few days of a bereavement, people can feel an urge to find distraction. It may be that something small or even banal – a pet's illness, a television drama or a rude salesman – will suddenly transport you away from the dreadful grief. It may be a drama in your own kitchen or the need to respond to a neighbour's generosity.

Almost anything that can distract a couple from their distress, if only briefly, is surely welcome. No one recommends drowning your sorrows in drink, but taking advantage of an unaccountable but positive change of mood can do no harm. We are often too hard on ourselves, too demanding, too solemn. There are no rules about handling grief, except perhaps, when you feel it, you should not hold back your emotions.

When a friend of ours went through a painful divorce, he found it both possible and strangely helpful to put on a quite different, jolly, persona when he went away at weekends from a London where everyone knew what had happened and expected only to see him in a distressed state. No one should feel guilty about these transitory escapes. One friend spent three months in total gloom after her fourteen-year-old son was killed, but was suddenly elated by lovely music from next door. Then she plunged into guilt at having forgotten her grief!

We would recommend not only distractions but deliberate

treats. When we were preparing for our only attempt at assisted conception, we promised ourselves that if it failed we should buy a charming Victorian folding chair we had seen that week in Hungerford. It still stands in our living room – rickety but evocative. If something eases the pain, feels right and harms no one, just do it!

Some find physical activity especially helpful, whether indoor or outdoor sports or simply shopping. Others go out for a meal, a film or discover a completely new scene – perhaps a railway trip to somewhere new, a weekend in Bruges, a coach tour of the Peak District, anything that lifts the eyes and mind from the gnawing pain within.

Couples may need to explore many different avenues, and not always the same ones as each other's. The man may be fortunate in his work, finding that he can 'forget' while he is concentrating on his job. On the other hand, it may be harder for him to encounter people with whom to share his grief. Some seek out a local men's support group, especially when the couple's relationship has been disrupted. Some find it easier to talk to strangers.

Needless to say, these roles may be reversed. If the woman's work is satisfying and the man is unemployed, his sense of failure and emotional isolation may become serious if not worked through and remedied. Likewise an increasing number of would-be mothers are single, older women who may feel particularly isolated when their grief goes unnoticed.

Compensation

Distractions are by definition spasmodic. More valuable are the genuine compensations that partly satisfy the couple's capacity for nurturing. Amid the early piercing griefs the idea of compensations may smack of bad taste, if not callousness. Yet the couple deprived of children gradually find consolation in their relationships with nieces and nephews or godchildren, or with the families of neighbours and friends. There may be times when a child will say, 'I haven't told Mum and Dad but . . .' and one realizes that the childless can have a role in being precisely *not* the parent.

As the Houghtons wisely note in their book on the subject: 'It can be a great privilege to be allowed a place in the lives of children and young people. Being a parent is [only] one way to take part in the human story . . . Each type of relationship has its own value.'[2]

Nevertheless there are limits to the closeness a non-parent can or even should achieve, and the child's parents may have feelings about this. Possessiveness can be a danger, as can spoiling the favoured child or becoming over-dependent upon the child's affections.

For some couples the company of other people's children remains more painful than rewarding. This may just have to be accepted. People have different needs and take different paths. Some will throw their energies into their paid occupation, others into voluntary work, pastimes or hobbies. Many partners will find new subjects for their powers of nurturing, and these need not be children. Helping adolescents can be especially rewarding but so can work with the adult disabled, the house-bound or old people. Others may find that the garden can absorb quite enough of their caring energies.

When couples are coming to the end of infertility treatment, it may be helpful for them to write down all the negative and all the positive aspects of their experience of trying to overcome infertility. They are often surprised how much they have gained in their ability to feel, express and share their emotions. Some have learned to be more assertive when dealing with authority. Some feel they have 'grown up'. One quoted an old Chinese proverb: 'It is better to light a candle than curse the darkness.'

Some of the childless are inspired to write more – perhaps joining a local writing class. Others prefer different creative endeavours such as sketching, painting, ceramics, flower arranging, carpentry, photography, cooking, drama or dancing.

Childless couples do, after all, have much more spare time than they were so recently expecting. However callous it may sound, there are significant advantages to not having children. Life without them is less hectic, less unpredictable, less fraught with anxiety, less expensive and, most obviously of all, much freer. The childless couple will not now become slaves to someone else's dietary, educational, entertainment and other needs. Nor will they bore their friends to the brink of somnolence by endless talk about playgroups and schooling. Their capacities for love and affection will generally need to be spread among different people and not concentrated within the family. They will have the maximum incentive to find a wide range of compensations and unexpected opportunities to enjoy them.

The couple may ask themselves whether they should use their freedom by fulfilling their old dreams of working overseas. They may consider helping a charity where there will be a deep sense of human need. As Diane Houghton movingly remarks of her own experience of childlessness:

Strangely, in entering the realms of the walking wounded, I feel that I have joined the mass of the human race. I have become aware that, in the balance of give and take over the past few years, I have had a very good bargain. I received much more than I gave. Now happiness seems less important than trying to understand. Now the giving has become less conditional.[3]

Part of a Larger Whole

This kind of mature acceptance may only come after many years. It may never come. Meanwhile a childless couple may have to cope with dozens of tactless remarks or clumsy assumptions that they never wanted children or were too busy or selfish to have them. Elizabeth was distressed by overhearing someone remark that she hadn't really wanted children because of her career (which was never the case). She was also upset to get letters from two women who had chosen not to have children and firmly assured her that childlessness would prove best. However painful this sort of behaviour is, the couple will recognize the need to adapt to their new circumstances. After all, one cannot always tell the insensitive person what hurt he or she is causing.

A bereaved mother who helps us at the MBF made a valuable point about this.

It may not be appropriate to direct one's response to the author of the hurt but it does need to be expressed. I remember receiving a very insensitive letter from a friend and as I read it I suddenly found myself feeling sick and faint and realized this was because I was trying to repress my (natural) emotional, hurt reaction. I think childlessness is a wound that heals but which remains as sensitive scar tissue which may bleed anew when something digs into it. When this happens, apply a dressing. Be kind to yourself and share it with someone who will understand and offer comfort.

Old feelings of grief, isolation, failure and perhaps anger are bound to reappear sometimes. Yet the murmurings of our more positive inner voices do gain strength as the years pass. Some of these may appear to be rather severe, but they need to be. A basic one runs something like this: 'Childlessness is tough. Life is tough. Now get back to it.' No one else should say, 'Pull yourself together,' but we might sometimes whisper it to ourselves.

The childless may need to beware of amplifying their loss with emotions transferred from quite other frustrations, regrets and losses from the past. All of us are capable of self-dramatization, or of projecting a deep-seated frustration about one problem – say professional failure – on to another like childlessness, where we might unconsciously sense a chance of receiving more ready, or less embarrassing, sympathy. A psychotherapist tells us she often sees people who have fallen into this trap whereby the new sorrow, perhaps the biggest yet, becomes still bigger and even overwhelming.

As we grow older, we will probably realize that childlessness is one of the many bereavements that occur to us. Life gives and takes away. We remember an old lady dying in a hospice, already half paralysed, partly deaf and wholly blind but now without pain and quietly cheerful. When someone dared to ask how she could be so contented, she smiled and said: 'God only lent me my legs, eyes and ears, and they were wonderful. Now I'm giving them back, one by one. That's only right.'

None of this is to deny the special pain felt by many among the childless in not having anyone uniquely to care for them in later years, whether in sickness, invalidity or old age, or to compensate for the eventual loss of their partner. Only a family continues to accept us more or less as we are. Nevertheless relatively few of the ageing can expect care within the family in our modern hyper-mobile society. Most old people, with or without children, eventually depend on professional assistance. A sort of ultimate childlessness may emerge as the fate of almost all of us. Some may see this as an aspect of a larger harmony in which life and death, receiving and giving back, are two faces of the same creative process.

One of the most moving of the many (anonymous) quotations from letters to the NAC that featured in the Houghtons' book is this from a man of eighty-eight who wrote in response to a radio broadcast in 1977:

Nobody has ever called me father or grandfather. I am now alone with the memories that other people pass on to their children. I am not afraid. I am a father, you see. Not to a person, but to those things I caused to be, the furniture I made, the people who relied on me. I wish you well with your association, but never make the mistake of believing the childless are not parents. All carry that love – there are many paths to follow.[4]

This is a perspective that unites both sadness and gladness within a wonderful transcending simplicity. It is one we ourselves hope to acquire as our remaining years pass by. It is the perspective of one who sees life and death whole, sees fertility and mortality in all its rich variety, and holds fast to intimations of a larger love.

We hope we have not generalized too much. In such a sensitive area individual responses can be so very different. A friend whose pregnancy ended in the miscarriage of her twin daughters wrote to us so movingly that we asked if we could quote her.

Obviously everyone has to find their own way forward. At the present my path, through what remains the most overwhelming disappointment of my life, is to take one day at a time and tell myself that, although I regret not knowing our children, not having been graced, as others are, by the mystery and magic of seeing one another's likeness and mannerisms carried forward into a future we shall not live to see, I do find meaning and fulfilment in the daily life we share. I have, after all, lived this much of my adult life without children.

With these small steps I am coming to see how my life is enriched in ways it would not have been had our children lived. Of course I would never have given them up voluntarily, but I recognize that children are a consuming passion, that the need to love and protect them uses up a vast amount of the love and energy that each of us has to give. Those of us who remain childless may pour that passion and concern into so many other aspects of life. It has taken me a while not to feel defensive about this freedom and to begin to appreciate and enjoy it, in its own right.

12. New Treatments and New Moral Dilemmas

Throughout history our notions about fertility, infertility and pregnancy have been compounded of myth, magic, lofty ideals and base prejudices – not least among clerics and doctors, nearly all of whom happened to be men. Some of their ideas showed ingenuity, even insight, but few bore much relation to women's experience or to what science has since learned. Dogma played a larger role than anything as mundane as observation. Nevertheless some of the ancient ideas still have a part to play, and sometimes a useful one, in the fervent debate about the rights and wrongs of the treatments available today.

One of the great theorists, Philip Melanchthon (1497–1560), believed the brain derived from pure semen. Nicholas Culpeper (1616–54) had the radical notion that the woman contributed to reproduction with an egg,[1] but conventional thinking, even that of William Harvey (1578–1657), persisted in attributing her with only a passive role. Such ludicrous ideas persisted well into the nineteenth century, when priests and doctors continued obstinately to defend their powers over women. None, for example, respected women's experience of quickening – the first sensation of the fetus moving inside the womb. And when it came to abortion – often euphemistically called 'expelling the termes' – the medical manuals recommended a bizarre assortment of herbal recipes, pessaries, bleedings, exercises, baths and purgative pills. Had men ever needed an abortion, the prescriptions would have been revised overnight.

Plato described the embryo as an animal. Aristotle thought the embryo passed through a plant-like stage, then that of a sleeping animal which later awoke in the womb. Male embryos, he believed, were formed and active at forty days; females took ninety. Aristotle believed that embryos already had souls, and this idea later shaped the Christian Church's stern views on contraception, paternity, abortion and other related issues. (The views of medieval Islam were often less rigid.)[2]

These great issues continue to fascinate and to divide us. What are we? How did we come to be? What determines what we are like? How did we grow? And what, most critically, is the moral status of the embryo, the fetus and the unborn child?

Contemplation of the mysterious origins of life can evoke ancestral fears of impiety and understandable moral disquiet as the development of infertility treatment appears to breach ever more taboos. The controversies surrounding the new developments can profoundly affect the feelings and decisions of the infertile and of their medical practitioners, let alone ordinary citizens, so it is important to explore these. Such debates can also affect the degree to which governments are prepared to fund new forms of treatment or, in some cases, to permit them at all.

Abortion as such is not our subject, but the perennial controversy about it is highly relevant to some of the core questions in the infertility debate, especially that of where (if anywhere) to put the 'great dividing line' between 'non-life' and life. Many people still think this is what should decide whether the manipulation, transfer or destruction of embryos is morally permissible. Others, as we shall see, contend that there can be no single physiologically or morally decisive line but several stages, each allowing a different moral judgement to be made.

In 1869 Pope Pius IX moved the dividing line back to what was called the 'moment' of conception. Abortion at however early a stage after conception became, therefore, the intentional killing of another human being – in essence, murder. This is still the official view taken by the Vatican, but it is contested by many within the Roman Catholic Church, let alone outside it. And, as we shall see, embryologists understand the subject altogether differently.

Rightly or wrongly, the preponderant opinion among the medical profession, women's groups and the liberal democracies in general, including people of every religious persuasion, is that abortion is legitimate when serious physical, emotional or social distress may otherwise be caused to either the child or the mother.

The Moral Status of the Embryo

The religious conservatives – Roman Catholic, Protestant, Islamic, or others – who see abortion as an evil, deploy the same basic principle of the sacredness of life to condemn both the fertilization of the egg outside the body (as in IVF) and the destruction of spare or rejected embryos that is often involved. They contend also that procreation should happen only in the act of love. In short, they say that the human soul should not be created in the laboratory and that the embryo has the same spiritual status and the same absolute right to life as any sentient human being.

There is another equally extreme but opposite view that is often stated with no less vigour and conviction. An eminent American geneticist told us he saw a fertilized egg in a dish as meriting 'no more respect than a smear of cells on a butcher's slab'. That this smear could be the beginning of a human life was, he said, merely incidental and 'the moral status of the embryo is nil'.

Many, perhaps most of us, would regard this view as an equally serious over-simplification. The cells in question already contain a full and unique set of human genes which could in principle create a Jane Austen, a John Donne or the butcher's only child. Yet to accord *some* moral status to the embryo is not to be forced to share the religious conservative's blanket opposition to assisted conception any more than their related condemnation of artificial birth control.

Supporters of the new procedures say that (as in the dilemmas over embryo reduction, discussed earlier) there is often an unavoidable need to make compromises between rival ideals. They argue, in particular, that the distress felt by deserving infertile couples must weigh more heavily than drily abstract principles about the embryo's allegedly absolute right to life or what is held to be 'unnatural' in procreation.

There is a clear parallel with the question of artificial birth control. Most people approve of it as one of the essential measures for relieving family poverty, infant mortality and the pressures of excessive population. They would therefore regard any 'principled' ban on the use of, say, condoms as not only indefensible but frankly immoral, considering how much needless suffering (not to mention AIDS) that these can prevent. Similarly its exponents see assisted conception as a vital means (within proper limits) of remedying the distress and psychological disablement of the unhappily childless.

Another moral puzzle here concerns the apparent inconsistency in the stand taken by the religious conservatives. Although they constantly insist on the absolute 'sanctity' of human life, they do not appear to adhere to this principle with anything like the same rigour in the context of war, as in the Vatican's doctrine of the 'Just War', or in relation to capital punishment, which it does not condemn outright. (Nor even does the Vatican absolutely exclude threats to use nuclear weapons.) The 'slippery slope' may apparently be encountered in the laboratory or clinic but not on the battlefield. Perhaps it may also be asked why, if the embryo is as sacrosanct as a developed human being, the Church does not treat the multitudes of dead fertilized eggs flushed away in lavatories with the same reverence as it does other departed souls?

We have no wish to upset Roman Catholics by posing these questions, but the Vatican's influence is strong, not least in the international community, as was evident in Cairo at the UN conference on world population and development (1994), and many people feel its present philosophy is as seriously misguided in relation to assisted conception as it is to artificial birth control and abortion. Liberal opinion is frankly astonished that distinctly questionable theological propositions are being put so far above the calls of charitable love, shared humanity and indeed the whole global outlook. Continued dialogue on these issues is plainly urgent.

Relatively recent embryological findings should illuminate this debate. For these seem effectively to dismiss the idea of a single 'moment of conception' (and hence a 'great dividing line') and reveal stages in the gestation of humans not wholly unlike those in the frog or butterfly. The fertilization of the egg is a necessary stage but so is the emergence of the primitive streak, the development of the fetus and then of the baby. If 'ensoulment' is to be thought of at all in this physical context, could it too not arise through a gradual process – including the acquisition of consciousness and intellect – rather than all at once?

An Ancient Tradition Meets Modern Embryology

It is fascinating to find that ideas like this – of stages rather than a 'great dividing line' – date back for at least two thousand years. There is a clear Western, and indeed Roman Catholic, tradition which maintains that the human embryo becomes animated by a rational soul at around forty days. Professor the Reverend G. R. Dunstan in his essay 'The Moral Status of the Embryo' describes how this idea was abundantly present in the writings of St Jerome, St Augustine, Pope Innocent III and St Thomas Aquinas.[3]

This creation of distinctions within the process of gestation was also present in early English statute law and remains embodied in Islamic law. In Roman Catholic canon law, however, it survived only until it was formally rejected, some say tragically, with Pope Pius IX's edict of 1869 (already mentioned), on the basis of which the Vatican still insists that the fertilized egg is itself already a human being.

Yet, as we have seen, recent research has given new grounds for rejecting this view. It transpires that until about fourteen days the 'embryo's' cells are undifferentiated, which is why it is sometimes described as the pre-embryo. At that time some of the cells migrate to form the so-called primitive streak (which becomes the embryo), while others become the placenta and its various membranes, which are also discarded at birth.

Many of the pre-embryo's cells, therefore, will not end up in the new individual. And not only may twinning occur; no fetus at all may be forthcoming. Instead the placenta may develop into a cluster of grape-like growths known as a hydatidiform mole. Or growth may just cease altogether. All this is good evidence for saying that individuality arrives not with conception but only with the primitive streak, when the cells migrate into specific positions ready for differentiation into tissues and organs.

The origin of identical twins sheds further light on this question. In the first few days after the egg is fertilized, a group of cells called the blastocyst develops and this then attaches itself to the uterus and becomes an embryo, then a fetus, then a baby. However, in the first fourteen days after fertilization, it can divide into two identical embryos. So the single blastocyst can – and quite often does – develop into more than one individual, and therefore more than one soul.

Indeed the blastocyst can go through one or more further splittings to produce identical triplets, quadruplets or even quintuplets. For example, the Dionne quins, the five identical sisters born in a Canadian farmhouse in 1937, came into being without any sort of medical interference. One 'conception' had produced not one soul but all of five souls, over several days.

A further illustration of the complexities of conception lies in the laboratory production of mouse chimeras. Black-and-white striped mice have been produced by combining in a laboratory dish the fertilized egg from each of two pairs of mice, one white-coated pair and one black-coated. Each of the resulting striped chimeras therefore possess the genetic material of *two* pairs of parents – four mice in all. If such a procedure was (outrageously) conducted with two human blastocysts, what were two potential souls would presumably have been merged into one. But at least this bizarre example shows that any notion of one key moment, one conception and hence, on the instant, one soul, is highly simplistic. And so, one would think, would be any dogmatic moral principle that is based upon it.

For Professor Dunstan, as for most philosophers, no moral agency or identity can arise without individuality; it is therefore at the stage of the primitive streak that he would attribute a status requiring protection.[4] But note that this does not mean that we have to give no protection to the pre-embryo or the early embryo, or total protection to the later fetus. In each situation there will be other moral claims of different weights to be placed in the balance. (This will become clearer when we discuss some of the more specific controversies.)

Pragmatic Doubts

Some people reject assisted conception for reasons not of allegedly overwhelming principle, as do the religious conservatives, but from disquiet about the present direction taken by modern medicine or by society in general. Some, for example, say medicine is over-emphasizing the needs of individual patients and neglecting public health (and preventive work), not least in the less-developed countries. Questions are raised, too, about over-dependency on the welfare state and our unwillingness to recognize that disease, frustrated hopes and death are ultimate features of life. Should we employ expensive medical procedures either to preserve life 'at all costs' or to produce new lives? Are we, it is asked, simply devaluing humanity's dignity and spiritual status?

One can sympathize with some of these fears without necessarily drawing the same conclusions. Modern medicine probably does tend to neglect the needs of society overall; to neglect older ways of healing, nurturing or consoling the whole person; and to encourage a new, self-interested health consumerism.

But to identify real or potential abuse is not to condemn assisted conception as such. The negative aspects of treatment must always be balanced against the remedying of the pain and destructiveness of infertility. For many people the inability to have children is a form of disablement worse than many more obvious ones. Moreover the procedures are not nearly as 'high-tech' or expensive as those employed in many other medical fields.

Those who oppose the notion of assisted conception but tolerate abortion seem especially hard to understand. Both interventions are deliberately interfering in matters of life and death; both involve no 'consent' from either the terminated or the created life. Both are intended to circumvent a serious situation in the life of the woman or couple. Should we not feel happier, if anything, to facilitate a conception than a termination?

A Brave New World?

One of the more particular charges laid against the reproductive revolution, as we mentioned at the outset, is that it is encouraging humanity to slide from procreation without coition ('babies without sex') to a eugenically controlled 'Brave New World' run by tyrants in white coats. Once we interfere in conception and gestation, we are told, full-scale genetic manipulation will follow and then the State will take charge of procreation to pursue its own dubious purposes.

It is true that we are already technically capable of selecting donors of ova and sperm in order to create or to exclude certain genetic qualities in our children, and that before long we shall be able to do this by choosing between various embryos created in vitro. We can also already identify the genes responsible for terrible conditions like Huntingdon's or Tay-Sachs (another inherited disease that causes brain degeneration and death) and are learning fast how to perform gene therapy.

Such technologies could plainly offer awesome possibilities to ruthless rulers following in the footsteps of Adolf Hitler, who attempted to create a 'pure' Aryan race by destroying Jews, gypsies, Slavs, the deformed and the mentally afflicted. It was therefore not surprising to read a recent *Sunday Times* headline speaking of the first steps towards creating a 'MASTER RACE'. At least in democratic societies, however, public alertness, the rule of law and professional standards will surely be strong enough to resist such extreme tendencies.

Commodification?

As we said in Chapter 2, some people are especially fearful of a growing 'commodification' of reproduction, whereby the child could become just another 'thing' to be purchased. Moreover, if not only IVF but gamete donation and surrogacy have prices put upon them, might not the commercialization of assisted reproduction become rampant? Certainly there must already be anxiety about the role of individual incomes in determining who gets what help. We return to this crucial issue of social justice in Chapter 14 when discussing the role of national health services.

In a Crowded World?

Infertile couples and infertility specialists are often bluntly asked whether there are not already too many babies coming into the world. It is a fair question. Human numbers have trebled in less than a century and the earth's fragile environment and finite resources are already severely strained. Some demographers fear yet another doubling of world population within fifty years unless radical action is taken.

Moreover the extra children resulting from assisted conception are mostly being born to the high-consuming and high-polluting societies of the rich North and therefore use up disproportionately more of the earth's resources at a time when the basic needs of the world's poor are being neglected. At least 300 million fertile women worldwide are said to want help with birth control but are unable to afford or obtain it.

To this the defenders of assisted conception say that against an existing annual population increase of 90 million worldwide, the addition of a few hundred thousand (or even eventually a few million) extra babies cannot be hugely significant. They say an anti-natalist policy, whether national, regional or global, cannot be seriously held to depend on the deliberate neglect of the infertile. The crucial issue is not what is to be done for the childless but whether the world community will pursue serious policies to foster population restraint, infant welfare, women's health and education and, not least, women's empowerment.

The sensible as well as humane approach is to help both the childless and the far greater number of couples who want to limit their family. Considering the scale of extravagance and waste in the world, we certainly have the means to do both, but this debate will clearly grow over the coming decades.

Feminist Fears and Hopes

Some feminists who deplore the apparent dominance of males and masculine perceptions in gynaecology are deeply suspicious of assisted conception. They suggest that men secretly envy women their reproductive powers and have a misogynistic dream of depriving women of their central individual role in procreation. Male doctors have also been accused of exploiting women's fears of being 'barren' to coerce them not merely into submitting to their clever new techniques but into craving them. Such feminists therefore argue that IVF can damage the woman psychologically by 'de-sexing' her and undermining her selfhood.

We have not ourselves encountered any IVF patients or mothers who talk this way. Nor have we met any of the infertile men who, allegedly, seek children via sperm donation so as to avoid the pains of undergoing treatment themselves.

In marked contrast other feminists welcome every step towards the mechanization of gestation, saying that only by taking reproduction out of the body can women become free. One writer has foreseen a pre-natal nursery in which unborn babies happily joggle together in a kind of giant aquarium.

Both these sets of views seem eccentric, even bizarre. A much more widespread feminist perspective sees the reproductive revolution of the 1990s as parallel to the contraceptive revolution of the 1960s in radically extending women's rights to control their own fertility. As Suzanne Moore stated in the *Guardian* (24 August 1994): 'The job of feminism should not be as a moral chaperone; it should be in the business of offering women as many choices as possible ... The problem here is not, as the detractors claim, that women are being offered too many artificial choices but that they are not being offered enough.'

Distortions of Moral Priorities

Taking this view, women – and of course men – are entitled not only to advice about infertility but to any necessary treatment. The neglected ethical issue is not that of technocrats manipulating embryos or extracting eggs from fetuses, but the failure of health services to do their proper job. If people are denied access to treatment through the NHS, can we be surprised that many will shop around, cut corners and even place newspaper advertisements for donor eggs?

People are also asking why so much moral debate is focused on single, lesbian or unmarried women rather than on the quality of parenting. Is there a distortion of our wider moral priorities when we worry so much about the 'designer babies' of tomorrow and so little about the 'off-the-peg' kind being born into grinding poverty every day?

Interim Conclusions

All these criticisms of the reproductive revolution deserve to be considered with respect, as they help us to recognize the manifold possible implications of each new stage. Nevertheless, some of the criticisms are put in such general or hypothetical terms that we are justified in putting greater weight on the more obvious and immediate benefits of assisted conception. But these, of course, must hinge on a satisfactory verdict on the greatest single issue: whether the children resulting from its procedures suffer physical or psychological harm as a result. As we said in Chapter 7, the results so far are reassuring, but we return to the subject in our last chapter.

The Libertarian's Challenge

Whatever general view any of us may take about assisted conception, whether as a doctor, health manager, politician, commentator, patient or ordinary voter, we are bound to ask ourselves how far we are entitled to impose that view on others.

The libertarian will say that ethical standpoints vary considerably, that none can be *proved* to be true and that many of the criticisms are not only pessimistic and speculative but rooted in unthinking revulsion at novel procedures. One journalist, for example, has written about 'artificially induced motherhood' reducing medicine to 'cannibalizing dead fetuses to create living babies'.

The libertarian's view accepts that some form of legal or other restraint is needed when there is clear danger of serious harm occurring to individuals or to society at large, but contends that we otherwise need to live and let live. Those who decry the new options should refuse to employ them, but leave others to make their own decisions.

Some people passionately disapprove of condoms, or even blood transfusions, but the rest of us justifiably insist on our own right to choose whatever does not seriously damage – and not just affront – others. It is too easy to be affronted, as many were by the first organ transplants, or to condemn medical innovations of which we ourselves expect to have no need. Moreover to ban something is not necessarily to stop it. No ethical or legal barriers will be effective unless there is general support for them. And practices banned in one country will probably be offered elsewhere, especially where big money may be involved.

Taken too far, the libertarian stance could lead to an extreme permissiveness, and a careful weighing of the implications of each new option is plainly vital, as we shall shortly see when discussing some of the more sensitive of the current controversies. Meanwhile, however, we should remind ourselves that for the infertile the new techniques constitute a wonderful extension of choice. Infertile couples not only accept but celebrate new opportunities for evading a cruelly childless fate. Some indeed see them as triumphs of humankind's God-given intelligence and creativity.

13. Current Controversies

The media have been bombarding us with ever more sensational stories about each new step in the reproductive revolution. They have rushed to tell us that someone has delivered triplets derived from her sister-in-law's eggs; that a Berkshire woman has produced four children by surrogacy; and that an Essex couple have – perhaps needlessly – paid to choose the sex of their baby.

A dozen editorials erupted when a Leicester man was said to be acting as a one-man sperm bank for single women and lesbians, and again when a research scientist in Washington, DC, claimed to have cloned human embryos (which could potentially enable us to create identical twins on demand). Especially widely reported was the British woman who had twins at sixty, following IVF treatment in Italy. Then there was the black woman who had obtained an egg from a white donor to reduce the chances of her child suffering racial discrimination. An exceptionally fierce storm raged when the work of an Edinburgh research team seemed to be making it possible to generate human eggs from aborted fetuses.

Some of our friends and colleagues have reacted with dismay, even disgust, to some of the newly emerging options. Others are worried about the 'unnaturalness' of the new procedures, or their social implications. Other people, though, are frankly delighted at the extension of medical potential and individual choice. Several of these anxieties we share, but sensible and widely acceptable conclusions will depend on a quiet examination of the detailed pros and cons, case by case.

This chapter will therefore examine some of the current

controversies before looking at which kinds of patient should be considered suitable for treatment.

The Shortage of Eggs and Embryos

A serious limitation on treatment for women unable to produce eggs themselves is the acute shortage of donated embryos and of eggs in particular. NEEDS estimated that in 1994 at least 1,500 women were waiting for donated eggs. To put this into perspective, only 407 women received eggs and only 82 were given embryos.

Eggs and embryos are also needed for research into infertility, genetic disease, the causes of miscarriage, the development of better techniques of contraception and methods of detecting genetic or chromosomal abnormalities in embryos before implantation. Unlike the religious conservatives, the BMA and the HFEA, for example, see no objection to these uses of the embryo up to fourteen days after fertilization – that is, before the appearance of the primitive streak.[1]

However, the issue what eggs or embryos from what sources are appropriate for transfer to patients, and on what conditions, presents a more difficult set of problems. Currently the main sources of donated eggs (and embryos) are those found to be surplus to IVF and GIFT treatments; eggs collected at the time of sterilization; and eggs donated by women purely for altruistic reasons. These sources were discussed in some detail in Chapter 5, as were the careful safeguards implemented in such cases. Three controversial new avenues are now being explored. First, the cloning of embryos; secondly, the grafting of ovarian tissue from the cadavers of young women; and thirdly, the development and transfer of ovarian tissue from aborted fetuses.

The Cloning of Embryos

In October 1993 Dr Jerry Hall of George Washington University reported success in dividing human embryos but had to stop his experiments within a week as a result of the hostile reactions he was receiving. He stated that his work was solely for research; yet it would in practice open up new, even bizarre, options for human reproduction. In late 1994, however, doctors at the Jones Institute in Norfolk, Virginia were reported (in the *Evening Standard*, 25 October 1994) as saying that they intended to clone embryos in order to assist couples in having a child or identical twins.

Cloning could well become a technically easy method of increasing the supply of embryos, but there are many objections to it, and especially to the use of such embryos in infertility treatment. Concealed physical harm could be done to them in the process of division. Clearly few people would approve of the deliberate production of identical twins for different mothers or for the same mother in different years. Even fewer would condone the creation of more than one copy of a human embryo, and the director of the Jones Institute has stated that he would not countenance this even though he knew it to be technically possible. As stated earlier, identical twins face special problems of identity: to create identical twins of different ages (or born to different parents) who did not know each other and without either's consent would surely be monstrous. It may be far-fetched to imagine a couple consenting to a copy of their embryo and hence their potential child being produced by another woman, but nothing is certain in this rapidly changing scene.

Yet cloning might be considered less controversial if the woman had produced only one egg and might not produce any more. It could then give her two or three embryos in what might be the last chance of an IVF transfer. Any resulting identical children would then at least be of the same age and have the same mother. (We will go into the British law on cloning in Chapter 15.)

The Use of Ovarian Tissue from Women

The grafting of ovarian tissue in animals has been carried out experimentally for about a century and has produced live offspring in mice, guinea pigs and sheep. The grafting of donated human tissue would probably be welcomed by women otherwise unable to produce their own eggs, even though genetically the eggs would be the donor's. (The same technique would allow a woman in danger of becoming sterile through cancer treatment to have her own ovarian tissue removed and later replaced.)

Different considerations arise about the use of ovarian tissue taken from a woman killed in an accident. She would certainly have needed to have recorded her consent to the use of parts of her body and specifically her ovaries. Her family might object independently to part of their 'blood line' being transferred to a stranger. But often the woman's family (and partner) will be relieved that some good should emerge from the tragedy.

Both these sources of ovarian tissue could in principle provide immature oocytes (eggs) to be matured in the laboratory, or ovarian tissue itself for grafting into women who needed it. A South Korean group has already reported its success with in vitro maturation of eggs obtained from donated adult ovarian tissue and the achievement of live births as a result.[2] This is not yet established medical practice and may not be generally approved by either the medical profession or the public, but research strongly suggests that transplanted human ovarian tissue, whether from the living or the dead, could well offer a source of eggs in the future. The BMA has envisaged a new category or organ being added to donor cards and these possibly being made available to girls of sixteen or even younger.

We see no insuperable objection to the use of ovarian tissue as such, granted proper consents and the absence of any commercial element or evidence of resulting harm on the children produced by this method. Following a six-month public consultation exercise conducted in 1994, the HFEA raised no objection in principle to the use of either eggs or ovaries from dead women but would not authorize the procedure in the UK until the problems of consent were further explored.

The Use of Aborted Fetuses: The Great 'Womb Robbing' Controversy

The use of ovarian tissue from aborted fetuses presents much greater problems on moral grounds and was opposed by the HFEA following the same consultation exercise in 1994 (in which 83 per cent of the responses proved hostile to the use of such tissue).[3] The possibility was little discussed until late 1993 when the press reported that Dr Roger Godsen at Edinburgh University had taken microscopic eggs from fetal mice, matured these in vitro, fertilized them and successfully implanted them into adult mice. It seemed plain that, one day, the same procedure might enable laboratories to create large numbers of human eggs.

The ovary from a fetus actually contains millions of immature eggs, whereas an adult donor, even after drug treatment, rarely produces more than twelve or fifteen eggs at a time. Alternatively, ovarian tissue from fetuses might be matured sufficiently in the laboratory for it to be grafted into a recipient woman in the same way as donated adult ovarian tissue.

The cries of 'womb robbing' have inevitably intensified. One

MP, Dame Jill Knight, found the idea 'absolutely revolting' – which she was entitled to feel – but called it 'Orwellian genetic engineering', which showed a basic misunderstanding of the procedure. She also told the House of Commons (on 12 April 1994) that 'it is wrong to get rid of an unwanted baby to make a wanted one'. This too misrepresents the question, since no one has suggested that abortions should be carried out *in order* to produce fetal tissue or that any commercial arrangement would be tolerated.

Her opponents pointed out that the use of some fetal material such as nerve, liver and pancreatic tissue has been sanctioned for some years under the Polkinghorne Committee's rules of 1989[4] and that fetal brain tissue, for example, was regularly used in the treatment of Parkinson's disease. Yet ovarian tissue and immature eggs can be seen to occupy a quite different category because they help create a new person and a continuing genetic line.

The arguments in favour of using fetal tissue mostly hinge on the urgent demand for more eggs and the risks incurred by women donors. Apart from the familiar absolutist objections raised by religious conservatives, there are some opposing arguments which are less familiar.

For example, some people object to creating life from a female human who never actually lived and could not 'herself' give consent. Others suggest that the eggs would be more likely to contain abnormalities than other donated eggs, although there is no special reason to think so. Some fear that the woman who had the abortion might claim 'grandmother's' rights over the resulting children, but regulations guarding anonymity would prevent this.

The most substantial objection to the procedure is once again that of potential psychological damage to any children produced, partly because they could have no mental or other image of a mother who never lived and partly because they might feel simple revulsion at their mode of origin. One critic has imagined possible cries of: 'Your granny killed your mummy before *she* was born!'

Plainly the rules governing the eventual use of fetal material in infertility treatment would need most sensitive drafting, including, as for other types of gamete donation, tight rules to prevent the occurrence of unwitting incest.

An Information Campaign?

Well before recourse is made to cloning or the use of fetal tissue or even the use of ovarian tissue from cadavers, there should be vigorous public campaigning on the needs of infertile couples, the shortage of eggs and how to help. There may have been official reluctance to pursue this policy as the demand for infertility treatment is bound to escalate when the egg supply improves.

Meanwhile some private clinics are reported to be providing free sterilizations or cheaper IVF cycles for women prepared to give eggs in the process. But this does not help couples who cannot afford private treatment and is anyway highly controversial. Some say it amounts to barter and hence is only commerce in disguise. Others claim it is acceptable granted proper controls concerning the health, anonymity and consent of the donor and the quality of the eggs.

Choosing a Child's Race

It is now technically possible for would-be parents to use IVF or GIFT as a tool for choosing the ethnic origin of their child by employing one or both gametes from selected donors. There is no interference with the genetic make-up of the gametes so, whatever else we may think, these are certainly not the 'designer babies' proclaimed in ignorant newspaper articles. Nor is it just 'consumerism'. To some degree, racial and other sorts of selection – for example, of 'blue blood' – has long been practised by royal families, among others, simply in the selection of the partner. A woman wanting a child of a particular colour has always been able to choose an appropriate father for her child.

The term 'racial selection' carries with it awful echoes of Nazi eugenics and, if widely practised, could become a socially explosive issue as well as being morally repugnant. Few, however, object if a Jewish couple want to adopt a Jewish child or an Italian couple wishes to avoid using a Nordic donor with ash-blond hair and Lutheran faith. The desire for physical and cultural compatibility seems unobjectionable and is certainly best for the psychological adjustment of the child. A black woman and white man would similarly deserve sympathy when declining the donation of an Asian or any other notably 'discordant' gamete. On this analysis the critical factors are not 'race' but compatibility and the psychological well being of the child.

In 1993 the Bourn Hall Clinic at Cambridge decided (with the parents' consent) to use a white egg when a black woman whose husband was of mixed race had waited in vain for four years for a black egg to be donated. (In Britain relatively few egg donors have emerged from among Afro-Caribbeans and people from the Indian subcontinent.) This decision caused a stir but seems entirely acceptable because, either way, a child of this couple would be of mixed race and hence compatible with the parents.

A less straightforward issue arose when a black woman, married to an Italian, deliberately chose eggs from a white donor in order to reduce her resulting child's 'blackness' and hence lessen any racial difficulties the child might encounter. It is not easy to condemn either the motive or the logic of this, which does put the child's interests first. But some people would see this as a step towards more sinister expressions of racial selection.

One philosopher, Professor John Harris, has been quoted as asking: 'Why should people not choose the race of their child by gamete donation when we permit them to choose their procreational partner?' Meanwhile other philosophers and theologians have said that such gamete selection is unacceptable because it 'objectifies' human life, treating children as if they were things.

Some see social selection of this kind as actually reinforcing racism, especially when particular racial characteristics are demanded. Many, however, believe it is a different matter when discordant characteristics are avoided because of the consequent mismatch between the parents and the child. The HFEA appears to take this view. It says the matching of donors should be carried out sensitively in discussion with the couples but that it would not be good clinical practice to allow a woman to choose for social reasons an egg donor of a different ethnic origin to herself or a sperm donor of different ethnic origin to her partner's. Libertarians, on the other hand, argue that couples should be able to make their own choices without interference from what they see as busybodies. Some ask whether a refusal to use gametes from different races is not itself a sort of racism by elevating race into a significant factor.

Choosing a Child's Gender

Many genetic diseases are sex-linked to male children and can therefore be avoided by giving birth only to females. The child's sex may be determined either by using 'female' sperm (in so far as these can be segregated) or by selecting a female embryo in the course of IVF. When employed for serious medical reasons, such action will not generally be opposed. An alternative would be to conduct an amniocentesis or equivalent test during the pregnancy and abort any male fetus. With naturally conceived pregnancies this is sadly the only practical alternative.

Some doctors claim already to be able to sort 'male' from 'female' sperm, but others doubt that this is possible. Timing of insemination is another but unreliable route, with selective termination in reserve if unsuccessful. Abortion on grounds of fetal sex alone is not permitted in Britain.

For couples to be allowed to select their child's gender for other than medical purposes, whether social, religious or economic, would be highly controversial and could have far-reaching consequences. Many people think the world shows quite enough gender prejudice, indeed outright misogyny, without new 'weapons' being added to its armoury. Women, families and communities could suffer badly if such sexist options were unleashed in Muslim countries like Saudi Arabia.

Yet there are arguments on the other side, and not just libertarian ones. Some parents who have had many children of one sex (like a family we know which has seven daughters) would give their eye teeth for a child of the opposite sex. Has individual need and freedom no claim in such cases? What harm could this do provided overall numbers of both sexes were roughly even? The gender balance is not affected if 'we' choose a boy and 'they' choose a girl. And might not the parents, happier at being given a choice, look after the resulting children better?

As to the wider picture, the demographic explosion hinges on the number of fertile women, not men, so arguably a pro-male bias would help slow down the rate at which the world population is expanding.

Again we reach treacherous moral terrain, where we feel torn between consideration of the freedom of individuals and the different consequences on society. A spread of gender selection might strengthen sexist tendencies in any society. It could also create new demands from normally fertile couples upon the limited resources available for IVF and GIFT, and further excite people's appetite for the more precise 'design' of progeny, even by genetic selection and manipulation. Despite such arguments the BMA's Special Working Party concluded in 1993 that, properly regulated, sex selection for social as well as medical reasons was ethically acceptable. This debate will clearly continue.

Male Pregnancy

Another potential debate is one so bizarre that we hope it will never receive serious consideration – that on whether men should be enabled to bear children. The idea of male pregnancy gained sudden currency with the release of the Hollywood comedy *Junior* in 1994, in which a character played by Arnold Schwarzenegger has a fertilized egg implanted in his stomach lining.

Although hormone treatments and new technologies (such as an artificial womb) may make male pregnancy possible, in no circumstances could we think such a development desirable or even tolerable. But no doubt some extreme libertarians will one day urge its acceptability.

Commerce? Anonymity? Consent?

Many of the other moral dilemmas currently hitting the head-lines have been discussed earlier in the book, such as those relating to commercial surrogacy (which is banned in the UK); the sale of ova and sperm; the uses to which frozen (early) embryos may be put; the anonymity of donors; and what limits there should be on the child's right to know about his or her origins.

Further highly convoluted issues are now emerging, for

which we have too little space. Such questions concern who has custody and who has rights over frozen ova, sperm or embryos when a couple have divorced or a donor has died. May healthy ova be taken from a seriously sick child to ensure that she may have a child later, if necessary by surrogacy? May a mother gestate her daughter's eggs? May the mother herself, though well past the menopause, insist on being implanted with her own eggs, frozen years earlier? And who has a right, and on what terms, to give or withhold consent for any particular procedure?

Who Should be Treated? At Whose Cost?

An especially sensitive group of issues concerns which kinds of women, men or couples should be excluded from assisted conception, whether by medical ethical committees, or even perhaps by law. (Who is entitled to get their treatment free is a different question, to which we come in the next chapter.)

The basic question here is whether anyone should be refused treatment if they are willing and able to pay. The answer must surely be 'yes'. A doctor would plainly be wrong to help contrive the birth of a baby for a couple of whom either partner was an alcoholic, a hard-drug user, prostitute, child abuser, mentally ill or HIV positive.

Some medical teams have declined to facilitate pregnancy in the blind, those confined to a wheel-chair or who are otherwise severely disabled. In such instances much depends on the partner and the wider context of the case, but candidates of this kind should be given sympathetic consideration as many of them have made excellent parents.

A fiercely contested question is what, if any, age limit should be imposed on women receiving treatment. After the sixty-year-old British woman gave birth to her IVF twins over Christmas 1993, it transpired that the Italian doctor concerned had successfully treated about sixty other post-menopausal women, although he was reported to have rejected over 400 women whom he judged physically unfit for such treatment.

Some people were thrilled for the 'granny-mothers', but more were worried about the outlook for the resulting children. The mother of sixty would be drawing her old age pension along with her children's allowance and would be at least seventy-five before her child left school.

For reasons of this nature few doctors would be willing to induce a pregnancy in anyone over forty-five or fifty when, for most women, fertility ceases naturally. Yet there may be special cases where a somewhat older but exceptionally healthy woman coming from a long-living family might reasonably be helped if she had a particularly supportive partner. No fixed age limit is likely to fit all cases and it would certainly be wrong to refuse treatment to women only because they were menopausal, for that may even happen in their twenties.

Some argue that if we are to have sexual equality and shared parenting, the age of the father should also be seen as relevant. Yet criticism of aged fathers is surprisingly rare: usually there are cries of: 'Isn't he wonderful!' Nor, so far as we know, has any age limit been suggested for the treatment of male infertility.

Is a Father Necessary?

It is often contended that medically assisted pregnancies should be available only to infertile heterosexual couples of normal child-rearing age who are living within a stable union. Indeed some authorities even insist that the couples should be married. But such restrictive notions do not take account of the wide variety of families that are now common, let alone the principle of people's freedom to choose the kind of partnership, if any, that they prefer. Many of the less conventional partnerships –

including some lesbian ones – are stable, happy and parentally successful. Many traditional married ones are not.

Difficulties almost inevitably arise for a single woman who wants a child but admits that she does not have a permanent partner. Some doctors would help her if she has good motives and her domestic situation is reasonably secure, and this is not forbidden by the HFE Act of 1990, despite its reference to the need for a father.

Single women have pointed out that over a quarter of today's families are brought up by single parents and that they generally make better parents than unhappy couples. Others insist that two parents of different sex is the ideal and that consciously to produce children lacking them is simply wrong. The participation of a father, or at least a second adult figure, is certainly desirable in bringing up a child, but insistence on any single criterion for good parenting is liable to lead to distorted conclusions in particular cases.

Clearly these cases can be immensely complex, and where there is a genuine dilemma a careful psychological assessment of the would-be parents is obviously essential. Any medical system has to beware of imposing dogmatic or perfectionist criteria of selection, bearing in mind that in the wider society there is virtually no control on who conceives by whom, with what motives or in whatever conditions. It would be absurd to demand impossible standards just of those who happen to be infertile. Moreover a doctor's prime responsibility is to his or her patients and their would-be children, and not to possibly prejudiced notions about the moral condition of the nation at large.

The HFE Act of 1990 rightly enjoins practitioners to exercise care in giving treatment where there is not a stable family background, and the Department of Health sensibly declines to define this term. Too many factors are involved. The Act also rightly requires doctors to take account of the welfare of any existing children – a need too often neglected.

Not only may a child have a different social and genetic father (such as a step-father or a male donor), we may have to ask whether there must always and necessarily be a living father, even at conception. Note, for example, cases where the wife of a dying man wishes to have his sperm frozen so that, even though she is to lose her husband, she is not deprived of her hope for their child. No one would say a consequent pregnancy was 'ideal', but how many would insist that such frozen sperm be destroyed at his death, notwithstanding his and her formally declared wishes?

The Need for Candour

Doctors recognize that people seeking treatment can be worried by so much talk of obstacles, but most clients present no great difficulty provided they are candid from the outset about any problems. Most medical practitioners will make their own appraisal of the patient's wishes, needs and circumstances, talk through the available options and seek genuine agreement on the wisest way forward.

14. The Debate about Public Provision for the Infertile

We hear a great deal from politicians and commentators about who they think should not receive infertility treatment, even when they can pay for it themselves. We hear much less about the far greater number of ordinary, desperate couples who should get treatment but don't. Many people regard the failure of Britain, and some other relatively rich countries, to provide free treatment as a much more significant moral issue than, say, the use of fetal tissue. This failure is actual, it is ongoing and it grievously affects tens of thousands of otherwise suitable candidates every year. It also raises fundamental questions about the sort of health service Britain has and what it ought to have.

It must be acknowledged at once that where time, money, skills and other resources are short, no single medical need can have absolute primacy. Somehow or other a society has to decide both the priority of different sorts of state expenditure, including health, and then its medical priorities as such. Most of us, for example, would agree that the claims of seriously sick children must take precedence over almost anything. Even though the childless may cry out, 'I have a right to a child,' we know that no such 'right' can be unconditional, as the most perfunctory thought about the poverty endured by the majority of the world's population will make clear.

The Provision of Infertility Services

The health budgets of most developing countries can provide only the very cheapest forms of infertility treatment, if any:

far too many of their most elementary health needs are still unmet. In these countries the World Health Organization inevitably puts much higher priority on life-saving procedures (and stresses the extra hazards attending multiple pregnancies).

By contrast, in many industrialized countries, including most of Western Europe, artificial conception is widely available at public expense, as described in Chapter 15. In France, Denmark, Belgium, Norway and Holland, for example, assisted conception is equitably available, either free or at very low cost. In Britain, however, there is still no national policy as such, nor even national criteria regarding suitability for treatment. Indeed discretion as to whether to give any free IVF or GIFT treatment at all is delegated to the many separate District Health Authorities. The result, as we shall see, is that most British couples without means are unlikely to obtain any treatment in assisted conception. Nor is such treatment usually available on medical insurance schemes, unless specifically contracted for – which few people could afford.

The availability of assisted conception is an issue of health policy that should concern not only doctors and health managers but every citizen. Opponents of free assisted conception often argue that infertility is not a disease and that life can proceed well enough without children for those so afflicted. Why, they ask, should expensive infertility treatment be provided when, for example, there are long queues for treatment of serious chronic conditions? What first are the facts?

Public Provision in the UK

A College of Health survey conducted throughout the UK at the end of 1992 established that 65 per cent of the District Health Authorities who responded (84.5 per cent in all) did not have a formal policy for the purchase of infertility treatments; 23 per cent were unable to give details of the specific treatments they bought for their patients; and 40.5 per cent of Health Authorities in England and Wales could not even say whether they bought treatment for ovulation induction. About 20 per cent explicitly said they did not buy IVF or GIFT treatments for their patients, but it seemed clear that most of the others did not do so either.

The survey also highlighted marked inequalities across the UK: geographical location often decided whether a patient could get treatment. (We have heard of a couple threatening to move home from Bradford to Leeds in order to improve their chances of receiving treatment.) Furthermore very different criteria were being applied: some Authorities defined infertility as one year of involuntary failure to conceive, while others specified four years. The definition of a stable relationship varied between one lasting two years (in south Cumbria) and four years (in west Essex). In some Authorities, IVF and GIFT were available only to women who were under thirty-five, or even thirty-four, at the time of referral, whereas others took women of up to forty-two years of age.[1]

A similar study conducted in 1993 produced some evidence that the use of formal criteria for treatment and the level of service purchased had increased. There was, however, no conclusive evidence of the latter and little to show that such money as was allocated to infertility was spent in the most cost-effective way. Some Authorities could provide no information at all about either the number of treatments of any kind offered in 1993/4 or of what would become available in the following year. A Department of Health report on hospital waiting lists that was published in November 1994 stated that, of the 524 patients who had been awaiting treatment for over two years, 523 – all but one, that is – were awaiting IVF.

In practice most parts of the British NHS currently provide few if any wholly free IVF treatments, even for highly suitable couples. (Such British District Health Authorities as are prepared to provide IVF or GIFT mostly expect couples to be childless, heterosexual, to have been living with their partner for at least three years and to be the kind of potential parent generally considered appropriate by adoption agencies. Some allow only one or two cycles of treatment.)

Nationally the actual levels of service provision and availability of infertility treatments have never been established but only a minority of Authorities seem prepared to pay for IVF or similar treatments at tertiary centres. One, in 1993, refused to buy IVF on the grounds that the treatment had only about a one-in-four chance (per cycle) of success and that the same money, put at about £2000, could purchase a new hip. (The same Authority was purchasing donor insemination at £70 per cycle. IVF produces more babies per hundred cycles than DI but its cost per birth is much higher.)

In 1992 a study at the University of Leeds calculated that, in an average health district with 250,000 people, around 230 new referrals to consultants for infertility investigations could be expected each year. These were estimated to produce 111 treatments and 30 live births, of which nearly a third would be low birthweight babies. All this would cost the district about £750,000 per year.[2] In 1994 a London Health Authority with over double the average population limited the annual amount it spent on fertility treatment to £150,000. It is not surprising, therefore, that about 95 per cent of couples receiving advanced infertility treatment are having to pay for it themselves.[3] Nor does this include the probably much greater numbers who could not afford to pay.

In the absence of nationwide (and even district and regional) figures for the annual number of infertility treatments given, and of what kinds and with what results, it is clearly not possible for the service to be adequately monitored, analysed or costed. This seems an extraordinary state of affairs and is scarcely consistent with the rhetoric of managerial effectiveness and rigorous cost-control that has surrounded the Conservative government's reorganization of the NHS.

The devolution of NHS decision-making to local Health Authorities, though in some ways useful, seems unlikely to bring much improvement. Financial pressures combined with local allocation of health priorities hardly favour the infertile, who, at a local level, tend to constitute a small, ill-organized minority. Thus any policy on infertility treatment that is fair, equitable and predictable seems bound to be one created on a national, not local, basis.

Allocating Medical Priorities

In Britain there are substantial and pressing medical needs that remain unmet, such as in the care of cancer and arthritis patients, the mentally ill and the increasing number of disabled elderly people. Should all such cases always take priority over the claims of the infertile?

One Authority we wrote to described the needs of the infertile as essentially social not medical. But the causes are indeed usually physical, and hence need to be treated medically, as do many of the consequences, like depression. Nor are the 'social' needs, if such they partly are, of necessarily lower overall priority than the medical ones.

In stark contrast to the stance taken by this Authority, Professor Richard Lilford, an infertility specialist at Leeds General Infirmary, was quoted in the *Independent* (11 May 1993) as saying that 'subfertility should have one of the highest priorities for NHS treatments and should come before chemotherapy for advanced cancers, before hip replacements and before cataract surgery.' He added: 'If someone asked me whether I would rather have a few more years of life or have my own children, I would have no hesitation in saying that children were more important.'

John Dickson, executive director of ISSUE, has been reported as saying that people received 'truly shoddy and rotten' treatment from the NHS, with little or no treatment being available in most parts of the country. He contrasted this with the considerable attention paid to the fertile majority who get every kind of help with family planning, contraception, abortion and sterilization.

We ourselves could not go as far as Professor Lilford, and believe only the most intricate assessment could determine which existing medical expenditures could reasonably be curbed in order to release funds to pay for assisted conception. Certainly, however, far too much is spent on excessive layers of management – of which we both have personal experience – and on questionable drug treatments, like tranquillizers. There is an urgent need for a comprehensive – not just local – reappraisal of how Britain is deploying its health budget.

As we have seen, many infertility treatments are both effective and by no means expensive. Some treatments using drugs to improve ovulation may cost under £100 per treatment. IVF treatment can certainly be expensive – at British private clinics it has been costing over £2,000 a try. Yet at one NHS clinic, at least, we have been told it currently costs them less than a third of that sum.

There are also allegations that in Britain many inappropriate and expensive treatments are given by family doctors or District Hospitals to women described as having unexplained infertility. Professor Robert Winston was reported as saying (in *The Times*, 20 October 1994): 'Money is being squandered. We are wasting huge sums. Every day women are getting hefty treatments of fertility drugs, costing up to £500, without even a proper diagnosis being made of why they are infertile. I saw five of them in my clinic yesterday.'

For reasons like this some specialists believe that the NHS's resources for assisted conception should be allocated on a more rationally coherent basis (based on centrally, not locally, determined criteria of need) and largely concentrated in relatively few supra-regional centres of excellence where expertise and facilities could be deployed more effectively.

Nor should it be assumed that failure to help those longing to have a family is itself without costs. As we have seen, infertility represents for many a deeply painful and genuine disability which can bring about mental distress, anxiety, grief, marital conflict, divorce, psychiatric illness and even suicide. All these possible consequences are a doctor's proper business and can themselves lead to high expenditure of both a medical and social nature.

There are some fundamental questions to be posed. Should a national health service be only a 'sickness' service? Is it not supposed to be concerned with the fullest functioning and well being of the whole person? For many people infertility not only frustrates a major purpose in life, it impairs their general happiness and, incidentally, their productivity.

Speaking of the reluctance of many NHS Health Authorities to provide adequate help, Polly Toynbee, the well-known BBC television reporter, has said (in the *Radio Times*, 21 August 1993): 'It's as if acquiring a baby were an optional consumer good, not an intrinsic part of human experience ... Some 600,000 couples could benefit from infertility treatment, yet health authorities are withdrawing from offering it.'

The normally fertile, including most health managers, tend perhaps to underestimate the extent and seriousness of infertility because it is still too often thought shameful and therefore not talked about. Many couples we know have never told us about their difficulties, despite knowing of our own experience and interests.

Studies in the US and Canada

Opponents of the free provision of assisted conception sometimes call in evidence the results of an elaborate process of assessment carried out by the American state of Oregon and implemented in 1994. Its authorities were rightly anxious to extend Medicaid coverage to residents who were below the US federal poverty line but, on a limited budget, this meant curbing the range of treatments that would remain available within the system.

A commission made up of doctors, consumers and representatives of the state's public health and social services therefore placed in descending order of priority over 700 medical services, with a view to eliminating those at the bottom of the list. Factors taken into account were effectiveness, the relationship of cost and benefit, data obtained from population surveys and public opinion assessed at local meetings.

Among the services ranked first were potentially fatal conditions, maternity care and preventive care for children. Infertility services were generally given low priority. IVF, as an expensive one, came only 696th out of 709 candidates.[4]

This was naturally a shocking finding for the infertile and the local professionals serving them. In an immediate outcry they stated that the survey method was biased because the large majority of people inevitably had little personal interest in artificial conception. They had either already had their children or had (so far) discovered no reason to expect difficulty or simply did not want a family. Everyone fears cancer or a bad accident: few expect to need IVF or are even especially aware of it.

In matters like this, much depends on the questions asked, and the context. Different findings emerged from a survey conducted on the subject for a report for the Canadian Royal Commission, published in 1993. Just over half those participating in the survey believed the costs of IVF should be shared between the couple and the government; a quarter of the respondents thought the couples should pay the full cost; and a tenth thought the cost should be met entirely by the public health insurance system.[5]

Fallacious Assumptions

Apart from its other failings, the Oregon exercise was based on the assumption that its existing health budget could not be substantially increased. This is frequently assumed in the UK too. The conventional wisdom is that medical budgets are finite but medical needs are infinite. Both these beliefs are open to challenge. The budget for any given year is bound to be limited and therefore to demand some allocation of priorities. But it is our political values and choices that decide whether that figure is too low or too high, not some remote objective rule as to what is 'realistic'.

The other conventional contention, that medical needs are infinite, has some superficial plausibility. It is undeniable that ageing populations and some of the rapid advances in medical practice are adding significantly to health costs. People are also more health conscious and more demanding. Yet medical needs are very far from infinite. Most people do not like being ill and have better things to do than trudge to the doctor, queue in hospitals or endure operations. Moreover, if medical demands are growing, so, mostly, are the advanced economies. Many will ask whether much of the annual growth could not be spent on health and education rather than on defence or on tax cuts that often most profit the better off.

Adherents of extreme 'free market' views frequently state that tax cuts are crucial to entrepreneurial incentive and hence a society's wealth, and therefore, in turn, its health and welfare provision. Sceptics may ask whether this is not an over-generalizing ideology which is of little practical value in determining what levels of provision are right. They pose a more pragmatic question, of whether inadequate health services are compatible with a fully productive let alone a contented society. They say Britain appears to spend significantly less of its gross national product on health than most West European societies, and that endeavouring to catch up with these countries could easily have closed most significant gaps in British health provision, including assisted conception for those needing it. Supporters of free provision also ask why, if revenues are so short, substantial tax reliefs are granted on house mortgages and various forms of share investment.

Critics of the current attitude towards health provision wonder why it tends to be thought of as somehow 'unproductive' expenditure, and suggest that much of it may be more sensibly regarded partly as real investment and partly as necessary insurance, rather than as 'hand-outs'. But more fundamentally they are questioning what they see as a grossly materialist philosophy that insists on seeing 'wealth' – and indeed 'reality' – as being essentially economic rather than also personal, social or environmental.

Campaigning for Help

Our concern here has not been to advocate any particular view of health economics but to show that the debate about it, and about free infertility treatment in particular, is far from dead. It will indeed intensify as the infertile organize themselves into pressure groups and as evidence accumulates of unnecessary waste and irrationality in other areas of public spending.

Meanwhile refinements in embryo culture, better equipment and improved diagnostic and treatment procedures are considerably reducing the cost of IVF and GIFT and improving their success rates. The studies of Dr S. L. Tan already show that, with IVF, women under thirty-four have comparable pregnancy rates to those of the 'normal' population. Both pregnancy and birth rates fall rapidly after thirty-five, but when donor eggs are used the live-birth rate for them is also high.[6] It looks as if increased expenditure would produce very satisfying results.

In Britain much depends on whether the infertility consultant at any given treatment centre is an effective lobbyist and whether there is a ground swell of opinion to which a District Health Authority can be induced to listen. Local champions are crucial, and women tend to be especially vocal in seeking proper provision. Perhaps the men should help more.

Opponents of free assisted conception sometimes allege there is very little support for it among family doctors. A study conducted in the Sheffield area resoundingly refutes this idea: a clear majority of the doctors surveyed were found to favour state-funded IVF and GIFT, let alone cheaper treatments; 58 per cent of them wanted no restriction on treatment to anyone under forty; 87 per cent said their local facilities needed increased funding.[7]

Critics of free treatment must also reply to the Royal College of Obstetricians, which has not only confirmed that the inability to have children can cause psychological distress and damage but that 'the pain of childlessness is every bit as great as that of osteoarthritis of the hip'.[8]

Looking Ahead

Difficult questions will always remain about which patients should receive IVF and how many attempts they should be allowed. Some Health Authorities are now devising and publishing their criteria for selection, so people will at least know where they stand. Public participation in such policy-making is permitted but underused. Community Health Councils could advise. Patients will not trust a system that does not listen.

There has been some good news, not least the growing hopes for cheaper treatments via 'transport IVF'. On this model, instead of the whole IVF process being conducted at the relatively expensive tertiary centres, the early stages such as investigation, counselling, hormone treatment and egg collection are carried out at cheaper 'satellite' units such as District Hospitals. When the time comes, the gametes are then swiftly transported to the tertiary centre for fertilization and embryo replacement. The NHS is thus spared expense and the couple much inconvenience. It should be added that some argue that the tertiary centres should in general be large, partly to gain the benefits of scale but also because their success rates are usually higher.

One report estimated that at least 275,000 infertile couples (in Britain alone) could be helped using this technique,[9] and one London unit reckoned in 1994 to have reduced the cost of an IVF treatment to about £580. The number of these satellite units offering transport IVF is increasing. A third of all licensed IVF centres are now involved in some sort of transport IVF. As this side of the work grows, the HFEA is rightly introducing new arrangements for its proper monitoring.

Some of the questions we have discussed in this chapter are personal as well as political, and we will all reach our own conclusions. But we hope to have offered some arguments with which to challenge the ill-informed and sometimes insensitive judgements responsible for the poor level of British public provision for the infertile.

15. Infertility Treatment and the Law

Not only individuals but electorates and governments take a close interest in any new procedures that can prevent conception, abort an unwanted baby, enable the childless to achieve a family or eventually affect the size or composition of a country's whole population.

But throughout history governments and churches, like individuals, have had deeper and more emotionally driven motives for seeking to influence sexual behaviour and reproductive activities. Over the centuries ruling opinion has tended to equate celibacy with grace, sex with sin and women with moral danger. Misogyny combined with prudery often induced those in power strictly to limit any interference with pregnancy or other 'natural' processes. Sometimes genuine reverence, caution and compassion played a part. Reproduction, sexuality and the role of the sexes are explosive subjects on which everyone has had their own views, and still do.

History

Issues of reproductive medicine first entered the British parliamentary agenda, and hence the statute books, in relation to abortion. Abortion is an unlikely, even cruel, subject for a book about infertility but it is inescapable because in Britain, at least, the law on infertility is rooted in the law on abortion. Morgan and Lee's *Blackstone's Guide to the Human Fertilisation and Embryology Act 1990* describes the background.[1]

Lord Ellenborough's Act of 1803 provided that the abortion

of a 'quick' fetus (usually defined as between the sixteenth and eighteenth week of pregnancy) was to be a capital offence. Abortion was sanctioned only where the life of the mother was at risk. In 1861 the distinction between abortions before and after quickening was dropped – along with the death penalty. But 'unlawful' abortion, variously defined over the years, remained and still remains a serious 'Offence Against the Person', whether committed by the woman herself or someone else. Further Acts followed. That of 1929 extended protection to the baby during the process of birth and to any fetus capable of being born alive.

The passage of the Abortion Act of 1967 left many of the previous provisions intact. However, it differed in two crucial points: it permitted abortion in certain specified circumstances and protected the medical practitioner, and the woman herself, from the 1861 offence of 'procuring a miscarriage'. There was of course massive public controversy over the moral principles involved, and medical, social and ethical argument persists over the definition of the terms 'abortion', 'miscarriage' and 'grave risk'. There is also still much dispute as to the age at which fetuses are 'viable', or 'capable of being born alive'.

The 1967 Abortion Act survived many challenges over the following two decades and then, in 1990, was recast in several ways by the Human Fertilisation and Embryology Act, upon which this chapter will focus. Apart from dealing with its main 'declared' subjects, the HFE Act amended the Abortion Act to reduce the time limit for authorized abortion from twenty-eight to twenty-four weeks. (Exceptions were allowed where the fetus had a serious abnormality or where the woman's health would be at risk.)

Background to the British Legislation of 1990

The Act, and hence the special Authority it created, came about only slowly but largely as a result of the 1984 Warnock

Committee Report, which appeared six years after the birth of the first 'test-tube' baby, Louise Brown. Then, in 1985, the Voluntary Licensing Authority (VLA), later to become the Interim Licensing Authority (ILA), was established by the Royal College of Obstetrics and Gynaecology and the Medical Research Council. By the mid-1980s the ILA had already approved thirty-eight IVF centres in the UK, of which seventeen were engaged in licensed research using surplus embryos or unfertilized eggs that had been fertilized **in vitro**. It had also established voluntary guidelines but these had no legal authority. This situation was plainly intolerable especially as a number of the clinics that had come into existence had been provided with inadequate equipment, staff and levels of supervision, and were producing unimpressive results.

During this period there was intense controversy, on the lines we have described, involving medical people and feminists as well as religious and other groups, as to whether IVF and embryo transfer treatments were sufficiently safe or efficacious, or even ethically acceptable in principle. When not only the successful but the failed treatments were taken into account, the true cost of each live-born baby following assisted conception was estimated in one American study in 1989 as at least US$40,000.[2] Other experts immediately joined battle, denying this flatly. But it was becoming evident to almost everyone who did not want these procedures to be banned outright that proper licensing and monitoring were essential both to control and to safeguard a rapidly burgeoning enterprise capable of great good but also great harm.

Some threats arising from the new technologies demanded early action, like the beginning of an international trade in human embryos for surrogate use. At that time there were also no legal limits or authoritative guidelines regarding the number of times a given donor's semen could be used to fertilize eggs. Hence there was some risk of producing unwitting incest not only between the resulting children but even between the donor and one of his own genetic offspring. (A Los Angeles newspaper reported that a man about to marry a much younger woman discovered she had been born following DI, so checked back for the time and place and discovered he was almost certainly her genetic father!)

With gamete donation it was also plainly vital to have adequate procedures concerning counselling and proper consents from both the would-be parents and the donor.

By 1990 there had already been cases where the fate of cryopreserved gametes or embryos had fallen into fervent dispute following a divorce or death. In Tennessee a custody battle broke out over seven embryos that had been stored prior to a marital break-up. The wife wished to use them to establish a pregnancy but the husband did not want her to have his child, or the child to be born into a broken home.

The judge had to decide whether the embryos were 'marital property' (to be divided equitably between the partners) or 'children' (to be passed to the better parent). He was reported as saying: 'I have absolutely no guidance, no direction, not only from the laws of this state, but indeed the world.' He finally awarded custody to the wife but this judgement was overturned on appeal.[3] Incidentally, British law does not recognize property rights in respect of human bodies, tissues or therefore embryos once they have been removed or stored. Thus if these are to be used in Britain, it can only be by the agreement of both partners.

In another case, after a rich Californian couple were killed in a plane crash and died intestate, the destination of a large bequest could have hinged on the fate of some cryopreserved embryos that might, through surrogacy, have produced new heirs. (A lesser question arising was whether such embryos could be used in research.)

The potential legal as well as moral complications arising from the new technologies were clearly multifarious and intricate. Practical experience showed that every case was different, so no dogmatic or unchanging set of regulations could possibly cover all of them. Furthermore to impose a rigid regime on doctors, clinics and research centres would destroy initiative, clinical freedom and flexibility of care. Such a system would be easier to police but every activity would have had to be covered in detail, making change well-nigh impossible. Both the HFE Act and the HFEA could have been brought into disrespect, perhaps contempt. A difficult balance therefore had to be struck between achieving a clear basic structure and real flexibility.

By the time the Bill was being debated in Parliament, many forms of assisted conception were producing many babies, many excited parents and many extravagant headlines, not to mention big business. Yet it was just not known how widespread the treatments were becoming nor what procedures or principles were being followed by which clinics. The hopes of some of the infertile were riding high, but the more thoughtful among them and very many health care professionals, moral philosophers and opinion-formers were becoming ever more fearful of poor standards, abuse of the treatments available and new unmonitored developments that might bring unpredictable and alarming results.

The financial, social and emotional costs of infertility treatments were exercising many minds. So, not least, was the rapidly rising number of higher multiple births and the distress these often entailed. In the *New Statesman* of 19 May 1990 one woman was reported to have suffered blindness, kidney failure and pleurisy at the end of a quadruplet pregnancy by GIFT. One of her quads died twenty minutes after birth, another at five months and the two survivors had multiple handicaps. It then emerged that she was not told about the possibility of a multiple pregnancy (let alone counselled about it) until a few moments before going into theatre for the GIFT procedure to take place.

Shocking stories were cropping up all over the world. The *Mail on Sunday* of 10 June 1990 reported that a woman in Western Australia, in whom IVF had resulted in quadruplet pregnancy, had vainly asked the clinicians to reduce the pregnancy to a singleton. Before the babies were born, she had decided to part with two or three of them and fourteen months later sent three of them for adoption, despite offers of financial assistance from the government.

There was, in short, increasing evidence that couples were not always receiving either the kind or the quality of care that they had a right to expect, that success rates were not always as good as they were made out to be and that considerable pain, distress and financial hardship were being caused.

Nor was the harm restricted to the would-be parents. Precious space in special baby-care units in the British state system, for example, were being taken up by a swift increase in the numbers of extremely small and premature babies produced as a result of multiple pregnancy following infertility treatment. Most of these, moreover, were coming from the private health system, without apparent regard either to the public purse or the interests of the singleton babies whom they often displaced.

Somehow, amid the raging arguments, a statutory scheme had to be produced that balanced the conflicting interests of many different patient, professional and other groups. These included the involuntarily childless who fervently wanted families; the children already being created by the reproductive revolution; the bearers of genetically inherited diseases or chromosomal abnormalities; and the donors of sperm or eggs where these were involved. Also included were the owners of infertility clinics already profiting from the new techniques; the scientists aching to get on with fundamental research; and religious and other critics of what they saw as profoundly objectionable manipulations.

The Act and the Authority

The HFE Act of 1990 was the first to put British infertility treatment and embryological research into a well-defined legal framework. Introducing it to Parliament, the then Health Secretary, Kenneth Clarke, called it one of the most significant measures to be brought forward by a government in the previous twenty years: it dealt with matters fundamental to the well being of society. In an earlier House of Lords debate, Lord Houghton had referred to it as 'a turning point in medical research and in the destiny of mankind'. As we shall see, these may not be exaggerations.

The need for legislation covering treatment centres, research clinics, storage places and the rights of all the people involved in treatment had become indisputable, and the HFE Act represented one of the first comprehensive set of measures the world had seen. Though not faultless, the British system still provides a useful – and adaptable – model for other legislatures to follow.

In essence the Act endowed the Human Fertilisation and Embryology Authority with real if necessarily circumscribed powers to regulate research on embryos, safeguard the integrity of reproductive medicine and give guidance to treatment centres on the standards and practice of good scientific and clinical practice. The Act was carefully framed so that the Authority could regulate work on infertility and genetic disease while resisting any Frankensteinian tendencies towards eugenics or other undesirable developments.

The HFEA is an independent body, funded partly by licensed treatment centres and partly by the taxpayer. Its work comprises the licensing and annual inspection of centres for treatment and research; the regulation of their activities, including the storage of frozen eggs, sperm and embryos; keeping confidential registers of donors, patients and treatments; giving advice to people seeking or providing infertility treatment; and constantly reviewing the whole field of both research and treatment.

The fertilization treatments covered by the Act, and hence the Authority, include only those involving the use of donated eggs or sperm (for instance, DI) and those in which embryos are created outside the body, as in IVF. It does not cover, therefore, surgical or other treatments of the causes of infertility in either partner, nor, for example, artificial insemination by partner, hormone treatments or GIFT (unless being carried out in a licensed centre).

The absence of any general regulation of GIFT is worrying. It is hard to understand why clinics providing IVF must be licensed and not those solely providing GIFT. The danger of producing high multiple pregnancies is no less great and the only difference is that GIFT does not involve handling an embryo as such. Many professionals regard this as a wholly insufficient justification for the exemption of clinics now practising GIFT but not IVF.

Yet GIFT treatment *is* regulated when donated sperm or eggs are involved – another evident inconsistency in the present arrangements. The HFEA must indeed license any clinic providing treatments of any kind that involve donor eggs or sperm.

For the many infertility treatment centres that do fall into the categories covered by the HFE Act there are detailed procedures of both licensing and regulation to ensure proper standards of equipment, safety, staff training, care and conduct, including the appropriate selection of women or couples for treatment. For example, the Act states that the centre must take account of the welfare of any resulting child (including its need for a father) and – very sensibly – of any other child who may be affected by its birth.

The Act gave the HFEA useful discretionary powers with which to develop detailed directives regarding many important areas, including the keeping of proper records of treatments and storage; the authorization of any payments to donors; requirements for donor selection; consents; and counselling. Other areas, such as research, are also covered and the resulting Code of Practice is regularly revised. Licences are only granted for limited periods, and teams of official inspectors – of whom Elizabeth is one – employ rigorous checklists.

Fees

Infertility centres and those involved in research and storage are charged licence fees by the HFEA, which has to raise 70 per cent of its income from such payments. A fee is payable for each IVF treatment cycle, a charge much resented by many practitioners and the infertile themselves. They say no other NHS (or private) treatment is 'taxed' in this way and that infertility treatment is already underfunded without further imposts being inflicted.

Advice and Counselling

In the HFEA's Code of Practice determining how the doctors select their patients, do their work and advise their patients, stress is laid on the provision of counselling. However, too few trained infertility counsellors are yet available and some private clinics resent adding to their costs by providing these. It is, nevertheless, vital to foster this side of treatment and to monitor longer-term outcomes, whether or not a baby results.

The lists of figures produced by the HFEA on the perform- ance of clinics are often said to be inadequate. Many people want some sort of league table to be published. The differences in both pregnancy rates and live-birth rates between clinics of similar size are still worryingly large, but achieving a fair basis of comparison may not be easy considering the wide range of patients' ages and problems.

Consent

People in general have a clear right to give or withhold consent to medical examination or treatment (unless, that is, they are unconscious or seriously mentally disturbed). Under the Act's Code of Practice, written 'informed' consent is therefore rightly required from the donor of eggs or sperm for either their use or storage, and from any woman using them. Clinics are also expected to acquire written evidence as to whether or not the woman's husband, if any, consents to the treatment or the gametes being stored. This may be important in any later dispute about the fatherhood of the resulting child. If the husband does not consent, the child may be legally fatherless.

A woman has the right to decide whether she agrees to all stages of IVF or GIFT treatment and how many eggs are to be used. She and her partner are also asked for written consent to the storage of their gametes or embryos, and to say what is to be done with them if either partner dies or becomes incapable. If the intention is that the stored materials should be donated to others, this has to be put in writing too. (The Code does not state what the storage authority should do if the parents say, for example, that their own children may use the gametes if they discover they are infertile or even decide in any case to generate their own genetic siblings.)

The Act's express prohibition of sperm storage without the donor's consent can lead to harsh results, as in the case of a young wife in 1992 who was refused permission to retain a sample of her husband's sperm when he went into a coma after a road accident.

Data Collection and Confidentiality

Apart from collecting material on treatment outcomes, the HFEA is required to register specific information on every IVF cycle and gamete donation and on the donors themselves. This is clearly essential for the proper supervision and assessment of the system.

As discussed at some length in Chapter 5, the HFEA has a legal duty to tell adults (who ask) whether they were born as a result of treatment using donated eggs or sperm. People aged sixteen or over can be told whether they could be related to someone they want to marry. Unless the donor's name and age had been recorded, no such assurance could be given. But it is important to appreciate that the donor's name – or other identifying information – cannot be disclosed. Indeed this would be a criminal offence except in rare cases – for example, where a child was born with a disability and wished to sue the donor as a result of the donor's failure to disclose a genetic disease. A specific court order might then require the Authority to make an exception.

Otherwise the Act does not itself indicate what information the children have a right to obtain: this will be up to the HFEA to regulate. Yet the HFEA does collect general information on what the donor looks like and gives him (or her) the chance to describe himself, including his interests and talents, and in his own words, if he thinks this might be helpful to a resulting child.

The Act does not absolutely prohibit the naming of the donor to the child but allows for Parliament, rather than the HFEA, to make new regulations about it in the future. However, any new decision on naming would not apply retrospectively – that is, not to earlier donors.

Aside from the Authority's own special if limited powers, the Act prohibits any licensee from divulging identifying information about either patients or donors to anyone not themselves covered by a licence, except in a few clearly defined circumstances such as where information is needed by medical staff involved in an emergency.

Research

The HFEA licenses research involving the creation of embryos in vitro or the use or storage of embryos. Licences are only issued if the project is thought necessary or desirable for specific purposes. These include promoting advances in infertility treatment; increasing available knowledge of the causes of congenital disease or miscarriage; or furthering the development of more effective contraceptive techniques or methods of detecting genetic or chromosomal abnormalities in embryos before implantation.

No human embryo may be kept or used after the appearance of the primitive streak. This is taken to be not later than fourteen days after the gametes are mixed (excluding periods when the embryo is frozen). Some researchers had hoped for a period of three weeks or more, and in some countries longer periods are allowed. Nor may a human embryo be placed inside any animal (or vice versa).

Licences may, however, be granted for performing 'the zona-free hamster oocyte test' for establishing the fertility of human sperm – which involves mixing sperm with the egg of a hamster – provided the resulting embryo is destroyed shortly afterwards.

Cloning

The cloning of an unfertilized egg may well prove impossible, what *is* possible is the division of fertilized human eggs to produce two or more embryos of identical genetic make-up — the resultant controversy was discussed in Chapter 13.

In Britain cloning by nuclear replacement — a sort of transplanting — is expressly forbidden by the HFE Act, but not cloning by splitting the embryo, provided that a licence has been obtained. The HFEA decided in 1994 not to license splitting embryos for purposes of treatment or for research to that end. Embryo biopsy is not barred provided that removed cells are not replaced in the womb. In no circumstances, however, may a human embryo be kept or used after fourteen days of development.

International Comparisons

The ethics, practice and control of various infertility treatments and of embryo research are being vigorously discussed throughout the world. In some countries any kind of embryo research is allowed provided there is no replacement of the embryo. In other countries some kinds of research, such as the creation of man/animal hybrids, are anyway prohibited. In countries where there is no formal regulation at all there may be some professional self-regulation, but it is in such countries that ethical boundaries are in greatest danger.

According to the survey by Gunning and English, there existed in 1993 no formal legislation on IVF or embryo research in Belgium, Canada, Greece (although an Act of 1992 paves the way here), Italy, Japan (where they are under solely professional control), the Netherlands (where regulation appears haphazard) or Portugal. Nor is there nationwide legislation in federations like Australia or the USA, or in Switzerland, where the cantons each have different laws about IVF but all ban research and surrogacy.[4]

It is worth mentioning some features of the system concerning embryo research and IVF treatment in countries which have passed controlling legislation. In Austria embryo research as such is barred but there are more reproduction clinics per million of population than anywhere else except Israel. A Danish Act of 1992 has provisions very similar to the British rulings except that they use regional ethical committees to oversee embryo research within the terms of the law. Treatment is available free in public hospitals.

The French ethical debate goes back to 1983 when a national ethics committee was established by decree. The Council of State then drafted a Bill in 1989 and an amended one was submitted to Parliament in 1992. In 1993 it had been put before the Senate when fresh controversy erupted, notably about cases of relatively old women receiving IVF. Sweeping bioethical legislation was passed in July 1994, but it avoided defining the legal status of the embryo for fear of giving ammunition to opponents of abortion for use in their campaigning. The question of whether embryos may be used for research therefore remained undecided.

IVF is very widely used in France, its cost being generally reimbursable by French social security. At the end of 1994 there were said to be about 20,000 surplus frozen embryos in storage.

The German debate is also longstanding, a commission on embryo research having been established in 1984. Consultation documents emerged in 1986 and 1988, and in early 1991 the Embryo Protection Act came into force. The Act is very restrictive and, for example, prohibits fertilization of an egg except for the purposes of pregnancy (and only for the woman who produces the egg). Cloning and the formation of human/animal hybrids are also prohibited, as is germline manipulation, which would alter the genetic composition of progeny. In all cases it is the practitioner, not those seeking treatment, who are liable. Over fifty centres undertake IVF but there is no regulatory body as such nor any central collection of statistics.

In Norway an Act of 1987 prohibits research (although this

is not closely defined) and limits IVF to married couples. Nor are donor gametes allowed in conjunction with IVF, and patients over thirty-eight are not treated. Surplus embryos may only be stored for one year, although many doctors seek an extension to three years. (The State pays 90 per cent of the cost of treatment at public hospitals and there is no limit on the number of treatments a patient may have.)

Spain was surprisingly early in setting up a commission and, in 1988, passing a law. This is comprehensive and extends to GIFT related techniques and DI as well as IVF. It is also perhaps surprisingly liberal in opening these services to any woman, married or not, and in allowing research on surplus embryos (up to fourteen days of development, as in the UK). The creation of embryos for research is forbidden, as is the freezing of eggs and any research involving cloning, parthenogenesis or genetic manipulation. The law also makes any surrogacy contract void. Treatment is available at many private and public centres – free at the latter.

The Swedish law on IVF came into force in the following year and is much less liberal. Couples must be married or in a permanent relationship. The use of donated eggs or sperm in IVF is banned, as is the donation of surplus embryos, and surrogate motherhood. Research is permitted only for the improvement of IVF techniques and no genetic or other manipulation of ova is allowed.

There has been much international discussion of these issues under the auspices both of the Council of Europe – for example, in its 1989 symposium on bioethics – and of the European Union. Neither, however, has yet achieved sufficient unanimity to draft any legal instrument or directive, whether on human rights, IVF treatment or embryo research.

16. The Priorities for Research

Governments become nervous when asked for increased spending on research let alone the health services, yet many people believe it to be equally important to direct new funding towards the diagnosis and remedy of disease as to spend it on building yet more roads or weapons of mass destruction. As we have shown, the human costs of remediable infertility are still widely underestimated; there is much still to learn and some areas of research have been seriously neglected.

The Psychological Impact of the New Technologies

The single most important focus for research must be the long-term outcomes for the resulting children. Evidence of either physical or psychological damage to the children – or to parents or donors – would clearly mean either improving or abandoning the offending procedures.

As we showed in Chapter 7, preliminary studies in the UK and Australia have been reassuring. They have shown no evidence of significant psychological damage to the children; indeed in some respects they reveal a better-than-average outcome. We must, however, await the results of several longer-term studies before concluding that the fears have been effectively groundless. The children will need to be twelve years old or more to understand and therefore fully react to some of the new methods that brought them into being. Nor is it inconceivable that some psychological damage would not become apparent until late adolescence.

Some psychologists fear that psychological damage could be done to children who are not allowed to meet their genetic parent – whether mother or father. Others are apprehensive about the potential effects on a child discovering it had sprung from the egg of an aborted fetus or a dead woman or a frozen embryo. One psychotherapist told us her mind boggled at all the possible implications and at the inevitable lack of experience of psychotherapists trying to help such patients.

Despite the good grounds for measured optimism, the monitoring of long-term effects on the children is essential for the reassurance of clients, medical staff, governments and the general public alike.

Should dependable evidence emerge of only slight damage to the children, an interesting question would arise. How would we weigh such evidence against the distress and damage suffered by the involuntarily childless? Do they too often think too much about their own needs compared to those of their potential offspring? We ourselves would think that the children's interests should remain paramount, and are worried by the sheer pace at which some treatments have been deployed.

Establishing Priorities

Further innovation in methods of investigation, surgery and treatment will clearly be pursued with enthusiasm and imagination, but work on methods of controlling and monitoring the impact of hormone treatments should be given particular priority because it is critical in reducing the numbers of higher multiple births and the great personal, social and medical costs to which these give rise.

The number of multiple births could also be reduced by improving methods of assessing the quality of embryos. If infertility clinics could transfer only one or two good embryos, they would not only cut the number of multiple births but reduce the IVF failure rate and hence also much distress, effort and waste of resources. It should also lessen the need for super-ovulation, with its various attendant risks.

The male factor in infertility, probably accounting for at least a third of all childlessness, also deserves greater attention. Far too little is known about its causes, let alone its remedies. Professor Dennis Lincoln of the Medical Research Council told the British Association at its 1994 conference that sperm counts in European men were falling by 2 per cent a year and in young men were significantly lower than in their fathers twenty years ago. A further set of important questions relates to the one-in-five cases of infertility that are from unidentified causes, not least those where both partners have produced children with earlier partners.

Environmental Dangers

In Chapter 4 we discussed the environmental threats to human fertility in relation to the possible impact of oestrogen-mimickers on sperm production. Investigation is also needed into many other disturbing occurrences in the natural world. In the Florida swamps, for instance, three-quarters of the eggs in some alligator nests are being found dead and many produce deformed offspring. In the Great Lakes of North America birds are suffering and many fish are unable to reproduce. This is also said to be true of many fish living below sewage outfalls in England. There are particular anxieties about the spread of pesticides, of the synthetic hormones present in contraceptive pills, of surfactants used in items ranging from detergents to cosmetics, and of dioxins resulting from the incineration of chlorine compounds widely used in the manufacture of plastics, solvents and paper.

In Britain the Water Services Association says there is a danger of people becoming unnecessarily alarmed and that soil or river pollution need not significantly affect actual water supplies. But if this is shown to be so, or if the oestrogen-mimicking pollutants turn out to be less destructive than is feared, there would be all the greater reason for wider-ranging research on the decline in male fertility. We suspect that this astonishing phenomenon will become a major preoccupation of the coming century and are ourselves amazed that it has so far evoked so little public and political interest.

Priorities for Prevention

It is far better to prevent infertility than to have to cure or circumvent it. Effective policies for prevention should tackle all the causes, whether environmental, nutritional, cultural, social, psychological or medical. To implement such a broad, holistic approach will cost money and therefore political choices. But the safeguarding of a nation's health, and the capacity to reproduce itself, is no small matter, quite apart from helping to lessen the distress experienced by countless individuals.

Expanded research into the causes of infertility will need to be accompanied by vigorous action, much of it necessarily international. If toxins are shown to be damaging the inhabitants of Europe, it would be no answer to export their chemical factories or poisonous wastes to dumping grounds in less-developed countries. Yet such cynicism is not unknown.

Among rich and poor nations alike, much research is needed into the whole epidemiology of infertility, not only its extent and causes but the effects of would-be remedies and of inadequate provision. Equally important is the preventive combatting of many known causes of infertility, including sexually transmitted diseases, IUD-related pelvic inflammatory disease, birth defects caused by certain drugs and various occupational hazards, as well as the environmental and other factors we have mentioned. While these subjects may not be the most scintillating from a medical point of view, they are, nevertheless, of special significance to poor countries.

Another matter of priority is an early reduction in the high number of back-street abortions, and this will require critical reappraisal of reactionary social policies; legal prohibitions on contraception as well as medical termination; and a review of some of the present religious teachings about sex, reproduction, gender and the family. The rights, dignities and welfare of women, including their education, civil liberties, employment status and political opportunities, are crucial. Their health and nutrition is also directly relevant to their fertility.

In at least twenty-five of the less-developed countries in Africa, Asia and the Middle East, the passage of girls into womanhood often involves cruel and harmful rituals. UNICEF says that more than two million girls each year suffer different forms of genital mutilation, which expose them to infection and ongoing reproductive problems. Such violations of elementary principle could be abolished under international conventions on the rights of the child.

In poor countries a combination of male prejudice in both the home and society at large leads to girls being substantially deprived of health care. Many more boys than girls are immunized. More are hospitalized when they are ill. A study of a Pakistani hospital conducted in 1990 found that 71 per cent of the children admitted under the age of two were boys. In many countries girls between two and five have higher death rates than boys of a similar age: in Haiti of every 1,000 such children 61 girls die compared with 48 boys. In the 'poor' southern nations, as opposed to the 'rich' northern ones, women do not generally live longer than men. One authority on the subject has spoken of 'the world's missing hundred million women': women who should be alive but are dead.

A Culture of Compassion

We have rehearsed what we regard as the chief priorities for research and preventive action, but it is no less necessary to foster a culture of compassion. Serious, and sometimes sacrificial, action will depend on motivation and feeling and political will, not just intellectual analysis. Such an outlook will, we believe, resist the rigid dogmatism of the religious conservatives but also the 'anything goes' enthusiasm of permissive individualists and over-ambitious researchers and practitioners. A mature approach will tread carefully, recognizing the moral claims not just of the prospective children but of the commissioning parents, the donors and surrogate mothers, the various medical and scientific professionals and of society at large. Only by promoting a culture of compassion that feels *with* as well as *for* all the people involved will we be able to avoid giving simplistic or dismissive answers to unavoidable and sometimes finely balanced dilemmas.

Assisted conception and its associated procedures can do great good, and stop great harm. They can also be abused. We were disturbed, for example, by a recent case that smacked of pure science fiction. An American woman was determined to give a child to her new husband but was herself, in her late fifties, well beyond egg-bearing. Her daughter therefore donated an egg, representing half of her own genes. This egg was fertilized in vitro with her husband's sperm and then implanted in a surrogate mother, who brought it to term. The resulting child thus had four parents occupying five different roles: the social mother, who had the original idea; a genetic mother (her daughter); a genetic father (the genetic mother's stepfather); a social father (who was also the genetic father) and a surrogate mother.

This is already a lot for the reader to digest, but note that the social mother was also her new child's genetic grandmother. Moreover the child's genetic mother (the egg donor) was also its half-sister.

Concern about assisted conception was reinforced in early 1995 with what the Italian press called an 'orphan birth' in a Rome clinic where the father's sister gave birth to his child using an embryo that had been stored before his wife's death in a car crash two years earlier (*Observer*, 15 January 1995).[1] In this case the resulting child was genetically wholly her parents' and the gestational mother was her aunt. Some might argue that an aunt is, if anything, psychologically preferable in this role than a stranger. Others see it as an intolerable emotional complication.

A further complication in the still developing saga of reproductive technology appeared in New York a week later when sperm was extracted from the body of a man killed in a fight, at the request of his widow (*Guardian*, 21 January 1995). On seeing his body the widow said she could only think about the children they had dreamed of having and asked for his sperm to be saved for use via IVF.

Yet another controversy loomed with press reports in March 1995 of 'Birth without Sperm'. Researchers at the University of Tottori, Japan, were thought to have fertilized eggs with vital genetic material isolated from the testes of men unable to produce sperm as such.

Such new possibilities may excite the imagination but they must sorely test the conscience. Our freedom has been enlarged but the dilemmas will not diminish.

Epilogue

Those of us who have not finally succeeded in having children will seek a mode of life that is creative and rewarding in other ways. But it will always be comforting to us if the fertile majority not only recognizes our enduring sense of loss but supports our call for increased medical help. Like us, the infertile still hoping for issue will need to raise their voices, but success will essentially depend on society as a whole hearing their call. The infertile need friends.

Despite all the complications, controversies and criticisms, we may surely celebrate the marvellous new ways of overcoming the fearful unhappiness of infertility. Perhaps yet another anonymous contributor to the *Prospect Newsletter* should be given the final word.

These days I am to be found attempting children's party cakes, cooking for fêtes and attending mothers' coffee mornings. Not quite the dynamic image of the nineties woman with brief case, mobile phone and filofax, but I absolutely love it . . . When the twins were about eight months old, I was playing with them one day, with the radio on in the background, when on came the same music I had heard in the theatre at egg collection time. It seemed to bring back the enormity [*sic*] of the miracle, and how very lucky we were that it worked. Just thinking about the tiny embryos we had seen on the screen, all contained in that little straw and then looking at our laughing gurgling babies, it just didn't seem possible. I started to sob with wonder and gratitude and all those sorts of feelings. So I turned the music up very loud, gathered up my babies and we danced around the room.

Notes

Chapter 2
1. G. R. Dunstan, 'The moral status of the embryo' in David R. Bromham *et al.*, *Philosophical Ethics in Reproductive Medicine* (Manchester University Press, Manchester, 1990), Chapter 1

Chapter 4
1. P. Patrizio and R. A. Bronson, 'The surprising male infertility – the cystic fibrosis connection', *Contemporary Urology* (June 1994), pp. 13–24

Chapter 5
1. *My Story* (Infertility Research Trust, Sheffield, 1991)
2. Robert and Elizabeth Snowden, *The Gift of a Child: A Guide to Donor Insemination* (University of Exeter Press, Exeter, 1993)

Chapter 6
1. P. J. Neumann, D. G. Soheyla and M. C. Weinstein, 'The cost of a successful delivery with in vitro fertilization', *New England Journal of Medicine*, 331 (1994), pp. 239–43

Chapter 7
1. C. E. Boklage, 'Survival probability of human conceptions from fertilization to term', *International Journal of Fertility*, 35 (1990), pp. 75–94
2. V. Beral *et al.*, 'Outcome of pregnancies resulting from assisted conception', *British Medical Bulletin*, 46 (1990), pp. 753–8
3. S. Golombok *et al.*, 'Quality of parenting in families created by the new reproductive technologies: a brief report of preliminary findings', *Journal of Psychosomatic Obstetrics and Gynaecology*, 14 (1993), pp. 17–22, and 'Families created by the new reproductive technologies: quality of parenting and social and emotional development of the children', *Child Development*, (in press)
4. H. Colpin and L. Vandemeulebroecke, 'The parent–child relationship

following in vitro fertilisation', presented at the tenth annual meeting of the European Society of Human Reproduction and Embryology (Brussels, 1994)

Chapter 8
1. C. Derom *et al.*, 'Iatrogenic multiple pregnancies in East Flanders, Belgium', *Fertility and Sterility*, 60 (1993), pp. 493–6
2. Merrel Pharmaceuticals Ltd, 'Clomid' in *Data-sheet Compendium* (London Datapharm Publications, London, 1981), p. 770
3. M. I. Levene, I. Wild and P. Steer, 'Higher multiple births and the modern management of infertility in Britain', *British Journal of Obstetrics and Gynaecology*, 99 (1992), pp. 607–13
4. P. A. L. Lancaster, 'International comparisons of assisted reproduction', *Assisted Reproduction Reviews*, 2 (1992), pp. 212–21
5. B. Botting, A. Macfarlane and F. V. Price, *Three, Four and More: A Study of Triplet and Higher Order Births* (HMSO, London, 1990)
6. Australian Multiple Births Association, 'Proposal submitted to the federal government concerning "Act of Grace" payments for triplet and quadruplet families' (Australian Multiple Births Association, Coogee, Australia, 1984)

Chapter 9
1. F. V. Price, 'Tailoring multiparity: the dilemmas surrounding death by selective reduction of pregnancy' in R. Lee and M. Morgan (eds), *Death Rites: Law and Ethics at the end of Life* (Routledge, London, 1994), Chapter 9, pp. 175–95
2. M. I. Evans *et al.*, 'Efficiency of transabdominal multifetal pregnancy reduction: collaborative experience among the world's largest centers', *Obstetrics and Gynecology*, (1993), pp. 61–6
3. M. I. Evans *et al.*, 'Attitudes on the ethics of abortion, sex selection and selective pregnancy termination among health care professionals, ethicists and clergy likely to encounter such situations', *American Journal of Obstetrics and Gynecology*, 164 (1991), pp. 1092–9

Chapter 11
1. Diane and Peter Houghton, *Coping with Childlessness* (George Allen & Unwin, London, 1984)
2. *Ibid.*, p. 144
3. *Ibid.*, p. 153
4. *Ibid.*, p. 144

Chapter 12

1. O. Thulesius, 'Nicholas Culpeper: father of English midwifery', *Journal of the Royal Society of Medicine*, 87 (1994), pp. 552–6

2. See G. R. Dunstan (ed.), *The Human Embryo, Aristotle and the Arabic Tradition* (University of Exeter Press, Exeter, 1990)

3. G. R. Dunstan, 'The moral status of the embryo' in David R. Bromham *et al.*, *Philosophical Ethics in Reproductive Medicine* (Manchester University Press, Manchester, 1990), Chapter 1

4. *Ibid.*, p. 6

Chapter 13

1. British Medical Association, *Medical Ethics Today: Its Practice and Philosophy* (1994)

2. Kwang Y Cha *et al.*, 'Pregnancy after in vitro fertilization of human follicular oocytes collected from non-stimulated cycles, their culture in vitro and their transfer in a donor oocyte program', *Fertility and Sterility*, 55 (1991), pp. 109–13

3. Human Fertilization and Embryology Authority, *Donated Ovarian Tissue in Embryo Research and Assisted Conception: Public Consultation Document* (HFEA, London, 1994)

4. The Polkinghorne Committee Code of Practice, *Review of the Guidance on the Research Use of Fetuses and Fetal Material*, Cm762 (HMSO, London, 1989)

Chapter 14

1. College of Health, *Report of the National Survey of the Funding and Provision of Infertility Services in the United Kingdom* (August 1994), commissioned by the National Infertility Awareness Campaign

2. 'Cost effective purchasing', *Effective Health Care*, University of Leeds, 3 (1993), pp. 10–12

3. P. R. Brinsden, '"Tax" on infertility is increased', letter in *British Medical Journal*, 309 (1994), p. 806

4. J. A. Kitzhaber, 'Prioritising health services in an era of limits: the Oregon experience', *British Medical Journal*, 307 (1993), pp. 373–7

5. Royal Commission on New Reproductive Technologies, *Proceed with Care* (Minister of Government Services, Ottawa, 1993)

6. S. L. Tan *et al.*, 'Cumulative conception and live-birth rate after in vitro fertilisation', *Lancet*, 339 (1992), pp. 1390–94

7. S. Thorton and I. D. Cooke, 'Should the NHS fund infertility services? A survey of Sheffield general practitioners' views', *Journal of Obstetrics and Gynaecology*, 12 (1992), pp. 353–4

8. Quoted in S. Redmayne and R. Klein, 'Rationing in practice: the case of in vitro fertilisation', *British Medical Journal*, 306 (1993), pp. 1521–4

9. C. R. Kingsland *et al.*, 'Transport in vitro fertilization – a novel scheme for community-based treatment', *Fertility and Sterility*, 58 (1992), pp. 153–8

Chapter 15

1. D. Morgan and R. G. Lee, *Blackstone's Guide to the Human Fertilisation and Embryology Act 1990* (Blackstone Press, London, 1991)

2. M. G. Wagner and P. A. St Clair, 'Are in vitro fertilisation and embryo transfer of benefit to all?', *Lancet*, 334 (1989), pp. 1027–9

3. J. Gunning and V. English, *Human In Vitro Fertilisation* (Dartmouth Publishing, Aldershot, 1993), p. 99

4. *Ibid.*, Chapter 9

Chapter 16

1. *Observer*, 15 January 1995.

Further Reading

Baruch, E. H., D'Adamo, A. F., Seager, J. (eds), *Embryo's Ethics and Women's Rights* (Haworth Press, New York, 1987)

Bartlett, J., *Will You be Mother? Women Who Choose to Say No* (Virago Press, London, 1994)

Botting, B., Macfarlane, A., and Price, F. V., *Three, Four and More: A Study of Triplet and Higher Order Births* (HMSO, London, 1990)

Bryan, E. M., *Twins and Higher Multiple Births: A Guide to their Nature and Nurture* (Edward Arnold, Sevenoaks, 1992)

Twins, Triplets and More (Penguin Books, Harmondsworth, 1992)

Dunstan, G. R., 'The moral status of the embryo' in David R. Bromham *et al.*, *Philosophical Ethics in Reproductive Medicine* (Manchester University Press, Manchester, 1990)

Freely, M. and Pyper, C., *Pandora's Clock: Understanding our Fertility*, (William Heinemann, London, 1993)

Gunning, J. and English, V., *Human In Vitro Fertilisation* (Dartmouth Publishing, Aldershot, 1993)

Houghton, Diane and Peter, *Coping with Childlessness* (George Allen & Unwin, London, 1984)

Jones, Maggie, *Everything You Need to Know about Adoption* (Sheldon Press, London, 1987)

Infertility: Modern Treatments and the Issues They Raise (Piatkus Books, London, 1991)

Leese, Henry, *Human Reproduction and In Vitro Fertilisation* (Macmillan Education, London, 1988)

Monach, J. H., *Childless: No Choice* (Routledge, London, 1993)

Morgan, D. and Lee, R. G., *Blackstone's Guide to the Human Fertilisation and Embryology Act 1990* (Blackstone Press, London, 1991)

My Story (Infertility Research Trust, Sheffield, 1991) – available from the Infertility Research Trust, University Department of Obstetrics and Gynaecology, Jessop Hospital for Women, Sheffield S3 7RE

Pfeffer, N., *The Stork and the Syringe: A Political History of Reproductive Medicine* (Polity Press, Oxford, 1993)

Pfeffer, N. and Woolett, A., *The Experience of Infertility* (Virago Press, London, 1983)

Royal College of Obstetricians and Gynaecologists, *Infertility Guidelines for Practice* (RCOG Press, London, 1992)

Royal Commission on New Reproductive Technologies, *Proceed with Care* (Minister of Government Services, Canada, 1993), 2 volumes

Snowden, Robert, *The Gift of a Child* (George Allen & Unwin, London, 1984)

Snowden, Robert and Elizabeth, *The Gift of a Child: A Guide to Donor Insemination* (University of Exeter Press, Exeter, 1993)

Spring, B., *Childless: The Hurt and the Hope* (Lion Publishing, Oxford, 1989)

Tan, S. L. and Jacobs, H. S., *Infertility – Your Questions Answered* (McGraw-Hill, Singapore, 1991)

Templeton, A. A. and Drife, J. O., *Infertility* (Springer-Verlag, London, 1992)

Winston, R., *Getting Pregnant: The Complete Guide to Fertility and Infertility* (Pan Books, London, 1993)

Glossary of Medical Terms

AIH artificial insemination by husband (*see* artificial insemination)

amenorrhoea the complete absence or cessation of menstrual periods

amniocentesis a procedure for identifying genetic disorders in the fetus from a small sample of amniotic fluid extracted with a special needle

anorexia nervosa a persistent refusal to eat, leading to serious loss of weight

anovulation the failure to ovulate

artificial insemination the introduction of sperm into the woman's genital tract by artificial means

azoospermia a complete absence of sperm

blastocyst a fluid-filled sphere of cells – a stage in the development of the zygote, four or five days after fertilization

blastomere one of the cells produced by the division of a fertilized egg

chromosome a tiny structure within each cell of the body, containing the genetic material that controls the functions of each cell

CISS computer image sperm selection (*see* p. 95)

clomiphene citrate a drug used to induce ovulation

corpus luteum follicle cells left behind in the ovary when the egg is released (*see also* progesterone)

cumulative conception rate a method of expressing the success of infertility treatment in achieving pregnancies which takes into account patients who discontinue treatment for some reason

cumulative live-birth rate as for cumulative conception rate, except for live birth rather than just pregnancy

DI *see* donor insemination

DIPI direct intra-peritoneal insemination (*see* p. 96)

DISCO direct injection of sperm into the cytoplasm of the oocyte (*see* p. 95). Also known as ICSI

donor insemination (DI) artificial insemination with donor semen

DOT direct oocyte transfer (*see* p. 94)

dysmenorrhoea painful menstrual periods

dyspareunia pain during sexual intercourse

ectopic pregnancy where the embryo becomes implanted outside the uterus, usually in the fallopian tube

egg donation the giving of eggs (oocytes or ova) by a donor to another woman

embryo a fertilized egg between two and eight weeks of development

embryo transfer transfer of the fertilized egg (or pre-embryo) into the uterus

endometriosis a condition in which endometrial tissue is found outside the uterus

endometrium the lining of the uterus which thickens during each menstrual cycle in response to the female hormones and is shed at the time of menstruation

epididymis a tightly coiled tube leading from the testis

fallopian tube one of two hollow tubes that project from either side of the body of the uterus towards the ovaries

fetus a fertilized egg from eight weeks' development up to birth

fibroid a benign growth of muscle appearing in the wall of the uterus

follicle-stimulating hormone (FSH) a hormone produced by the pituitary gland in response to LHRH, released by the hypothalamus. It stimulates development of the ovarian follicles

FSH *see* follicle-stimulating hormone

germ cell the sperm or the egg

GIFT gamete intra-fallopian transfer (*see* p. 93)

Gn-RH gonadotrophin-releasing hormone (*see* LHRH)

gonad an ovary or testis

gonadotrophin a hormone that stimulates the testes or ovaries – e.g. follicle-stimulating hormone (FSH) or luteinizing hormone (LH)

gonadotrophin-releasing hormone (**Gn-RH**) *see* luteinizing hormone-releasing hormone

HCG *see* human chorionic gonadotrophin

HMG *see* human menopausal gonadotrophin

HSG *see* hysterosalpingogram

human chorionic gonadotrophin (HCG) a hormone extracted from the urine of pregnant women and used to trigger ovulation when the follicle has reached an appropriate (pre-ovulatory) size. It is the hormone measured in the pregnancy test

human menopausal gonadotrophin (HMG) a hormone extracted from the urine of post-menopausal women and used to induce ovulation in women not responding to clomiphene citrate

hydrosalpinx a swelling at the end of a blocked fallopian tube

hymen a thin membrane surrounding the opening of the vagina that is usually broken at the first intercourse

hyperprolactinaemia excessive production of prolactin

hyperthyroidism excessive secretion of thyroid hormone

hypogonadism/hypogonadotrophic a condition whereby the pituitary gland secretes insufficient gonadotrophins to stimulate the gonads

hypopituitarism underactivity of the pituitary gland

hypospadias incomplete development of the penis

hypothalamus the part of the brain which secretes luteinizing hormone-releasing hormone (LHRH)

hysterectomy the surgical removal of the uterus

hysterosalpingogram (HSG) an X-ray test involving the injection of dye into the uterus to enable examination of the uterine cavity and fallopian tubes

hysteroscopy an inspection of the inside of the uterus using a telescopic instrument

ICSI intra-cytoplasmic sperm injection (*see* p. 95). Also known as DISCO

impotence the inability of a man to have an erection of sufficient firmness to perform coitus and impregnate his partner

intra-uterine insemination the injection of sperm directly into the uterus through the cervix

in vitro fertilization (IVF) the fertilization of the egg by the sperm in a dish before transfer to the womb. Popularly known as 'test-tube baby' treatment

IUI intra-uterine insemination (*see* p. 96)

IVF *see* in vitro fertilization

IVF-ET in vitro fertilization and embryo transfer (another term for IVF)

IVM in vitro maturation of oocytes (or eggs)

Klinefelter's syndrome a congenital abnormality causing male infertility, in which a man has an extra X (female) sex chromosome

laparoscopy a method of examining the pelvis whereby a laparoscope is inserted into the abdominal cavity and attached to a light source

LH *see* luteinizing hormone

LHRH *see* luteinizing hormone-releasing hormone

libido sex drive

luteal phase the second half of the menstrual cycle after ovulation has occurred and the corpus luteum is formed

luteinizing hormone (LH) a hormone that is produced by the pituitary gland and stimulates the final maturation of the egg

luteinizing hormone-releasing hormone (LHRH) a hormone released by the hypothalamus that stimulates the pituitary gland and ovulation. Also known as gonadotrophin-releasing hormone (Gn-RH)

luteinizing hormone-releasing hormone analogue a compound in which the chemical structure of natural LHRH is slightly altered

MAF micro-assisted fertilization (*see* p. 95)

MESA microsurgical epididymal sperm aspiration (*see* p. 96)

micromanipulation procedures for helping the sperm penetrate the hard outer covering (or zona pellucida) of the egg

multicystic ovaries a condition in which the ovaries are enlarged with cysts

oestradiol one of the three oestrogen hormones produced in women

oestrogen the female hormone produced by the ovaries

oligospermia a condition in which too few sperm are produced

ovarian hyperstimulation excessive stimulation of the ovaries

ovary one of two organs which contain the eggs and produce hormones, mainly oestrogen and progesterone

pelvic inflammatory disease (PID) infection of the pelvic organs (uterus, fallopian tubes and ovaries)

PID *see* pelvic inflammatory disease

pituitary gland a gland that is located at the base of the brain and produces many hormones, including follicle-stimulating hormone (FSH), luteinizing hormone (LH) and prolactin

polycystic ovary syndrome a condition in which the ovaries become filled with many tiny cysts that interfere with menstruation and ovulation and may cause obesity, acne, greasy skin and unwanted hair

POST peritoneal oocyte and sperm transfer (*see* p. 94)

pre-embryo a term previously applied to the human conceptus in the first fourteen days of its development. The term 'embryo' is now more commonly employed

premature ejaculation the ejaculation of sperm before the penis enters the vagina

primitive streak a stage in embryonic development when the cells start to migrate before forming specific organs

progesterone a female hormone produced by the corpus luteum after ovulation

prolactin a hormone produced by the pituitary gland

PROST pronuclear oocyte stage transfer (*see* p. 94). Also known as ZIFT

pulsatile LHRH therapy a method of administering LHRH at regular intervals to mimic the normal pattern of hormone release from the hypothalamus

PZD partial zona dissection (*see* p. 95)

semen the fluid, including sperm, released at male orgasm

seminal vesicle a male 'accessory gland' that produces some of the seminal fluid

seminiferous tubule one of the tiny tubes in the testes in which sperm develop

speculum an instrument used to examine the cervix and vaginal walls

spermatogenesis the process by which sperm are produced

split ejaculate a method in which only the first part of the ejaculated sperm is used for assisted conception

surrogate a fertile woman who has a baby (often produced by one or more donors) which she hands over at birth

SUZI sub-zonal insemination (*see* p. 95)

TET tubal embryo transfer (*see* p. 94). Also known as TEST

TEST tubal embryo stage transfer (*see* p. 94). Also known as TET

testis/testicle one of the paired sex glands which produce sperm and testosterone

testosterone the male hormone produced by the specialized Leydig cells within the testes

TUFT trans-uterine fallopian transfer (*see* p. 95)

Turner's syndrome a congenital abnormality in which a woman has only one, instead of two, sex chromosomes and is usually infertile

unexplained infertility a diagnosis made after full investigations fail to reveal the cause of infertility

urethra the duct by which urine (and semen in the male) is expelled

uterus the womb

varicocele a collection of dilated 'varicose' veins in the scrotum that may be associated with infertility

vas deferens the convoluted duct that carries sperm from the testis to the ejaculatory duct of the penis

ZIFT zygote intra-fallopian transfer (*see* p. 94). Also known as PROST

zona pellucida the tough, outer covering of the egg

zygote a fertilized egg of up to about fourteen days' development

Where to Find Help: Some Useful Addresses

British Agencies for Adoption and Fostering (BAAF)
Skyline House
200 Union Street
London SE1 0LY
Tel (0171) 593 2000
Fax (0171) 593 2001

British Association for the Betterment of Infertility and Education
PO Box 4TS
London W1A 4TS

British Homeopathic Association
27A Devonshire Street
W1N 1RJ
Tel (0171) 935 2163

British Infertility Counselling Association (BICA)
The White House
High Street
Campsal
Doncaster DN6 9AF

British Organization of Non-Parents (BON)
BM Box 5866
London WC1N 3XX

CHILD
PO Box 154
Hounslow TW5 0EZ
Tel (0181) 571 4367

Childlessness Overcome Through Surrogacy (COTS)
Loandhu Cottage
Gruids
Lairg
Sutherland
Scotland
Tel (01549) 2401

DI Network
PO Box 265
Sheffield S3 7YX

The Endometriosis Society
35 Belgrave Square
London SW1X 8QB
Tel (0171) 235 4137
Fax (0171) 235 4135

Family Planning Association (FPA)
27–35 Mortimer Street
London W1N 7RJ
Tel (0171) 631 0555
Fax (0171) 436 3288/5723

The Human Fertilisation and Embryology Authority (HFEA)
Paxton House
30 Artillery Lane
London E1 7LS
Tel (0171) 377 5077
Fax (0171) 377 1871

Institute of Psychosexual Medicine
11 Chandos Street
Cavendish Square
London W1M 9DE
Tel (0171) 580 0631

ISSUE
(formerly the National Association for the Childless – NAC)
St George's Rectory
Tower Street
Birmingham B19 3UY
Tel (0121) 359 4887

Miscarriage Association
18 Stoneybrook Close
West Bretton
Wakefield WF4 4TP
Tel (01924) 484515

Multiple Births Foundation (MBF)
Institute of Obstetrics and Gynaecology
Queen Charlotte's and Chelsea Hospital
Goldhawk Road
London W6 0XG
Tel (0181) 740 3519/3520
Fax (0181) 740 3041

The National Egg and Embryo Donation Society (NEEDS)
Regional IVF Unit
St Mary's Hospital
Whitworth Park
Manchester M13 0JH
Tel (0161) 276 6000
Fax (0161) 224 0957

National Infertility Awareness Campaign
99 Bridge Road East
Welwyn Garden City
Hertfordshire AL7 1BG

Parent to Parent Information on Adoption Services (PPIAS)
Lower Boddington
Daventry
Northants NN11 6YB

Progress
(the campaign for research into human reproduction)
27–35 Mortimer Street
London WC1
Tel (0171) 436 4528
Fax (0171) 637 1378

Royal College of Obstetricians and Gynaecologists
27 Sussex Place
Regent's Park
London NW1 4RG
Tel (0171) 262 5425

STORK
(the association for families who
have adopted children from
abroad)
Dan Y Craig Cottage
Balaclava Road
Glais
Swansea SA7 9HJ

**Twins and Multiple Births
Association (TAMBA)**
PO Box 30
Little Sutton
South Wirral L66 1TH
Tel/Fax (0151) 348 0020

Wellbeing
(the health research charity for
women and babies)
27 Sussex Place
Regent's Park
London NW1 4SP

Index

READ MORE IN PENGUIN

In every corner of the world, on every subject under the sun, Penguin represents quality and variety – the very best in publishing today.

For complete information about books available from Penguin – including Puffins, Penguin Classics and Arkana – and how to order them, write to us at the appropriate address below. Please note that for copyright reasons the selection of books varies from country to country.

In the United Kingdom: Please write to *Dept. JC, Penguin Books Ltd, FREEPOST, West Drayton, Middlesex UB7 0BR*.

If you have any difficulty in obtaining a title, please send your order with the correct money, plus ten per cent for postage and packaging, to *PO Box No. 11, West Drayton, Middlesex UB7 0BR*

In the United States: Please write to *Consumer Sales, Penguin USA, P.O. Box 999, Dept. 17109, Bergenfield, New Jersey 07621-0120.* VISA and MasterCard holders call 1-800-253-6476 to order all Penguin titles

In Canada: Please write to *Penguin Books Canada Ltd, 10 Alcorn Avenue, Suite 300, Toronto, Ontario M4V 3B2*

In Australia: Please write to *Penguin Books Australia Ltd, P.O. Box 257, Ringwood, Victoria 3134*

In New Zealand: Please write to *Penguin Books (NZ) Ltd, Private Bag 102902, North Shore Mail Centre, Auckland 10*

In India: Please write to *Penguin Books India Pvt Ltd, 706 Eros Apartments, 56 Nehru Place, New Delhi 110 019*

In the Netherlands: Please write to *Penguin Books Netherlands bv, Postbus 3507, NL-1001 AH Amsterdam*

In Germany: Please write to *Penguin Books Deutschland GmbH, Metzlerstrasse 26, 60594 Frankfurt am Main*

In Spain: Please write to *Penguin Books S. A., Bravo Murillo 19, 1° B, 28015 Madrid*

In Italy: Please write to *Penguin Italia s.r.l., Via Felice Casati 20, I–20124 Milano*

In France: Please write to *Penguin France S. A., 17 rue Lejeune, F–31000 Toulouse*

In Japan: Please write to *Penguin Books Japan, Ishikiribashi Building, 2–5–4, Suido, Bunkyo-ku, Tokyo 112*

In Greece: Please write to *Penguin Hellas Ltd, Dimocritou 3, GR–106 71 Athens*

In South Africa: Please write to *Longman Penguin Southern Africa (Pty) Ltd, Private Bag X08, Bertsham 2013*

READ MORE IN PENGUIN

A SELECTION OF HEALTH BOOKS

When a Woman's Body Says No to Sex   Linda Valins

Vaginismus – an involuntary spasm of the vaginal muscles that prevents penetration – has been discussed so little that many women who suffer from it don't recognize their condition by its name. Linda Valins's practical and compassionate guide will liberate these women from their fears and sense of isolation and help them find the right form of therapy.

Mixed Messages   Brigid McConville

Images of breasts – young and naked, sexual and chic – are everywhere. Yet for many women, the form, functions and health of our own breasts remain shrouded in mystery, ignorance – even fear. The consequences of our culture's breast taboos are tragic: Britain's breast-cancer death rate is the highest in the world. Every woman should read *Mixed Messages* – the first book to consider the well-being of our breasts in the wider contexts of our lives.

Defeating Depression   Tony Lake

Counselling, medication, and the support of friends can all provide invaluable help in relieving depression. But if we are to combat it once and for all, we must face up to perhaps painful truths about our past and take the first steps forward that can eventually transform our lives. This lucid and sensitive book shows us how.

Freedom and Choice in Childbirth   Sheila Kitzinger

Undogmatic, honest and compassionate, Sheila Kitzinger's book raises searching questions about the kind of care offered to the pregnant woman – and will help her make decisions and communicate effectively about the kind of birth experience she desires.

The Complete New Herbal   Richard Mabey

The new bible for herb users – authoritative, up-to-date, absorbing to read and hugely informative, with practical, clear sections on cultivation and the uses of herbs in daily life, nutrition and healing.